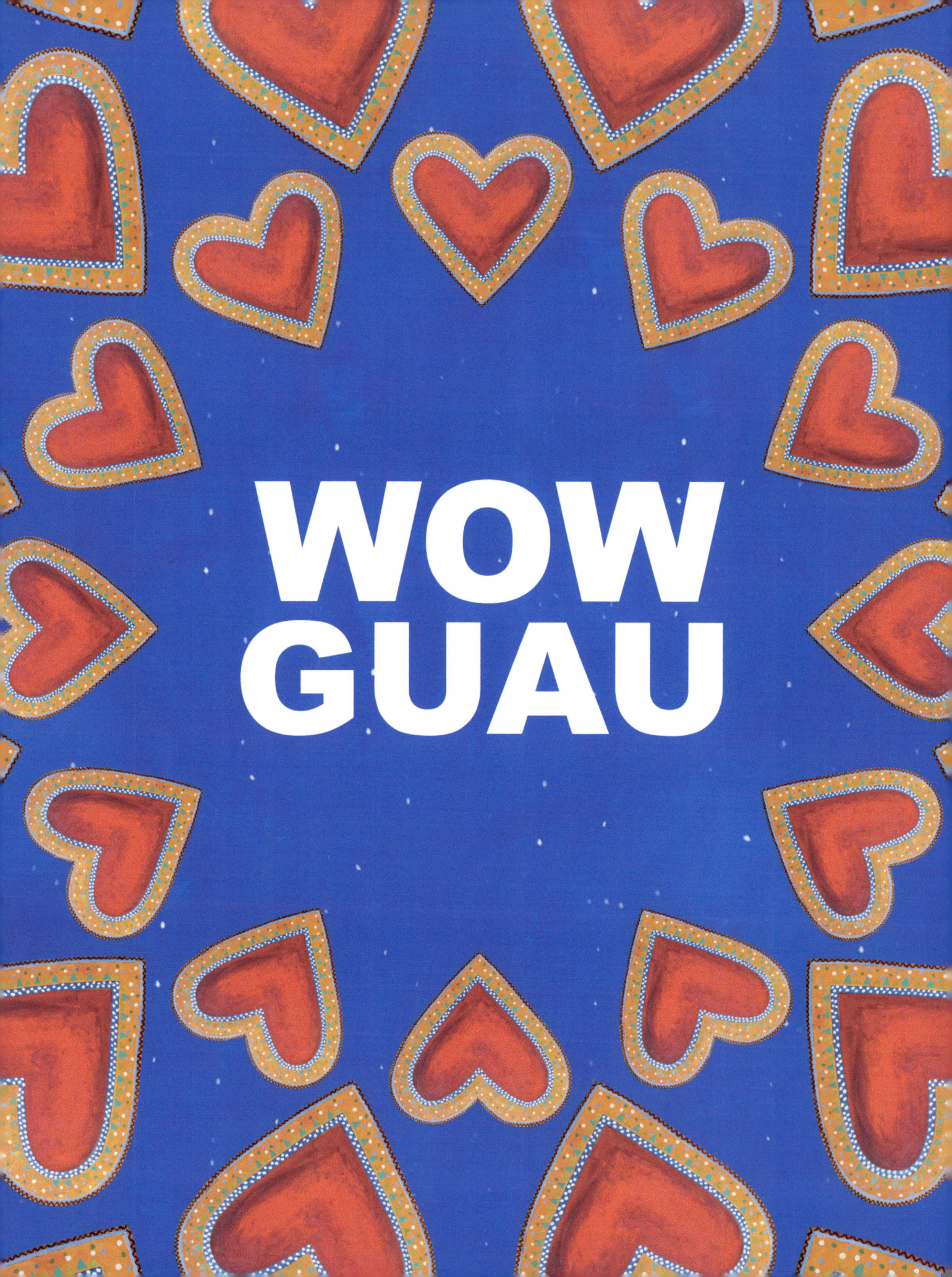

WOW of the Magical Body

...an unusual reference book of the human form, geometry and its connection to the universe.

By: Nanette E. Hayles

This book is dedicated to ALL those who have searched and are searching and will search for TRUTH.

Question... Are you a human body having occasional spiritual experiences or are you a spiritual being experiencing what it`s like to have a human body?

Partial Answer: When you are asleep, do you know if you are a man or woman, human or a plant, Jewish or Palestinian, from Mars or Earth, hungry or full, educated or ignorant, black or white, Hitler or Buddha? Think about it.

COPYRIGHT © 2018 by Nanette E. Hayles
Derechos © 2018 por Nanette E. Hayles

WOW of the Magical Body /GUAU del Cuerpo Mágico

Library of Congress United States (con derechos internacionales en Mexico)
Biblioteca del Congreso de Estados Unidos.

All rights reserved, including right to reproduce this book in portions there of in any form whatsoever, without prior written permission of author.
Todos los derechos reservados. Esta publicación no puede ser reproducida en su totalidad ni en partes, en ninguna forma o ningún medio sin previo permiso escrito por el autor.

Note: Author encourages Fair Use with proper acknowledgement of author and those in the biography. One is encouraged to use and share brief portions of the information contained in this book including drawings for spiritual and educational purposes only. (Not for sale, reprint or distribution purposes).

Nota: El autor alienta el uso correcto con su debido reconocimiento y los de la biografía, se recomienda que use y comparta partes breves de la información contenida en este libro, incluidos dibujos con fines espirituales y educativos únicamente. (No para fines de venta, reimpresión o distribución).

Available ebooks English version: IBSN 987-0-9986666-2-4 Ingram Spark
First Publication 2019: Ingram Spark POD (print on demand) books IBSN 978-0-9986666-3-1
Printed in USA

Disponible libro electrónico en Español: Ingram Spark IBSN 978-0-9986666-4-8
Primera Publicación 2019: Ingram Spark IBSN 978-0-9986666-5-5
Imprimir E.E.U.U.

WOW of the Magical Body

Continue your experiences from "WOW of the Hearts" to "WOW of the Magical Body".

In "WOW of the Hearts" you have learned a way to still your mind and how to live more from your heart. With these *tools* of listening to your own heart's wisdom and voice, we can apply what we have learned and continue our knowledge with "WOW of the Magical Body". We will travel through our own bodies and find out what each part does. Through our journey we will discover its magic and its connection to geometry and the world. With this knowledge we can awaken our innate abilities and actively participate in our bodies' functions, which can directly improve and maximize our health and lives. This is also an integral step in healing our spirits and our planet.

Table of Contents

Part 1 Sacred Geometry Basics and how it relates to life and the Human Body

    Phi Ratio: The Blueprint of Life (One Dimensional Line)   13
    Fibonacci Sequence   13
    Fibonacci or Golden Spiral (Three Dimensional Plane)   14
    Golden Means Rectangle (Two Dimensional Plane)   15
    PHI Ratio of the Human Body Form   16
    Creation Manifests:
        1. First 7 days: Genesis / Flower of Life   17
        2. Egg of Life, Seed of Life and the Fruit of Life   18
        3. Flower of Life (extended)   18
    Creation Continues to Manifest: the Elements
        1. Metatron's Cube   19
        2. Platonic Solids   20
        3. Pillars of Life   21
    Universal Language Math and Geometry   22
    DNA, Health and Epigenetics   22

Part 2 Glands of the Endocrine System of the Human Body

    Adrenal Glands   27
    Gonad Glands (male and female)   29
    Pancreas Gland   31
    Thymus Gland   33
    Thyroid Gland   35
    Parathyroid Glands   37
    Hypothalamus   38
    Pituitary Gland   39
    Pineal Gland   40

Table of Contents

Part 3 Organs of the Body
    Brain: Nervous System   43
    Heart: Circulatory System   45
    Lungs: Respiratory System   49
    Liver: Digestive System   50
    Spleen: Lymphatic System   51
    Gallbladder: Digestive System   52
    Stomach: Digestive System   53
    Small Intestine, Large Intestine (Colon, Rectum, Anus): Digestive System   54
    Kidneys: Urinary System   57
    Bladder Ureters and Urethra: Urinary System   59
    Reproductive System:
        Female organs: vagina, clitoris, vulva, uterus, cervix, breasts   60
        Male organs: penis, testicular sacs, prostate   61
        Procreation   62

Part 4 Frequency Waves (Hertz) and Light Waves (nanometer) Spectrums
    Total (known) Spectrum   67
    Our Spectrum   67
    Frequency, Wave Length and Proton Scales   68
    Colors, Musical Scale and Emotions   69
    Vibration and the Spectrum in Human Emotions   70
    Matisse Finds a Way   71

Part 5 Ancient Schools of Wisdom
    Kabbalah and the 13 Sephiroth   75
    Three Pillars of Life   84
    Inverted Tree of Life   86

Part 6 Addendum to Book 1, Wow of the Hearts: 90
    Practices to do along with meditation   91

Foreword

"We are in a process of unlearning...a crucial and necessary step for it creates a space for Truth."

The purpose of this book is to explore, expose and empower the magic of our bodies and its other connections. "Wow of the Magical Body" is for everyone and it is more than just a reference book. It will continue to answer questions as we grow and develop, supplying knowledge to our mounting curiosities. It is obviously not the answer to all questions, as the body is a highly complex organism, subject to the environment and its etheric/aura, mental, emotional and spiritual fields. This book will present various perspectives for your consideration that can help you maneuver through the information and give you a better understanding of the body and some of its interesting aspects. Some may find this book a bit controversial because I have taken the liberty to connect dots that many people, living in the box, would not consider connected or related. These connections, I have discovered, make our human forms as well as all of creation more magical. The PHI ratio for example is one of those connections. This ratio exists in all of nature. Historically, PHI is basically known through artists and architects that have copied this blueprint source and utilized it in some of their own creations. But the PHI relationship was known and used thousands of years before recent artists and architects revived PHI and made it more known to the public. The famous great Pyramids of Giza in Egypt and Solomon's Temple are just two examples of the ancient use of PHI. In our more recent history, the paintings of Leonardo Da Vinci and some of the modern architecture of I.M. Pei reflect knowledge and use of PHI.

I have also attempted to provide other ways of thinking that empower and promote health. One of these ways is to reconsider the following, that the physical disease or illness that happens to the body is usually and actually the manifestation or the effect of something else that caused that illness. Illness is actually the result of not addressing or listening to that something from a specific area of the body or mind that is trying to get our attention. The cause is almost always manifested by the deeper more primary illness that existed within the emotional and mental auric fields of our physical form. Illness originates in the mind and or in the emotions first: it is the point of origin. It then manifests physically in the body. Illness does not happen the other way around, matter then mind. The mind-thought blueprint vibration of the illness is first, before the actual physical manifestation of the illness.

This way of thinking and approaching illness is becoming more commonly accepted in the West. Disbelief or dismissal of this possibility may cause cognitive dissonance where the mind may not want to reconsider other ways illness can manifest. Instead, we continue to hold on to the present notion of the origin of illness. However, please reconsider and relax the mind, take a breath and let another way enter your consciousness. Play with the new idea and imagine the possibilities surrounding it. These battles of cognitive dissonance, of stretching our mind or expanding our mind to open up a bit more to other ways of thinking, can actually be moments of profound realizations. We will find that when we imagine, more possibilities exist.

We can then utilize and integrate more of our own higher faculties in deciding which ideas seem plausible, workable, useful and more fulfilling and which ones do not. This process promotes inner growth and validates further investigation within Self, the place where all answers truly and ultimately lie. We will discover that these moments can be our greatest triumphs in expanding our consciousness; exposing and opening us to a path that can help us remember and discover more of who we actually are.

This project took almost five years and originally it was a reference book that would define and show the body's parts and their relationship to the basic chakras, but it evolved into something much more than the original vision. As I investigated alternative studies of the body, as opposed to the mainstream broken and fix-it approach, I knew I had to include the PHI ratio, the Pillar of Life, frequency, the Inverted Tree of Life and the Kabbalah and its 13 Sephiroth. Each aspect studied empowered my inner will not only to understand, but to also experience some of the new revelations of these studies. Portions of the book had to be rewritten as my clarity and understanding evolved. Intuitively I felt that with each connection, there was a light revealing another deeper aspect of the same truth. Some of the connections to truth exposed are that there exists a basic order to things or matter, a structure or laws that are molds for the *sculptures* of life. We can choose to be in harmony with those laws or choose otherwise. Another truth re-exposed is the dualistic nature of this 3D Earth realm. We must realize and accept that for now we do not have control over this aspect of life. But we can and do, right now, have control over ourselves. Our world can and will change only when we individually and collectively evolve. The ancients offered us a way out, a way to maneuver through the swing of the pendulum, the to and fro of polarity that is prevalent in this world.

The Kabbalah offers a way out or way *inward* from the constant bombardment of the swing through teachings that empower one, not to change the world, but to change one's self; to evolve and transform one's energy and one's frequency so that it resonates in the realm of the higher emotions of understanding, appreciation, forgiveness and compassion. The Sephiroth each represents another aspect of who we are and the power we each possess is already within us. To awaken it we must have the desire, the drive and the will to want IT, the reconnection to the Divine. Otherwise, we are subject to polarity and its swing of the pendulum. Through establishing equanimity we find a solid ground in which to reconnect our auric fields of body, mind, emotions with spirit, improving not only our own personal health, but contributing to the overall health of our collective family. I hope some of these alternative ways presented in this book will be considered and used in your own personal investigation of Self and all that the self encompasses. It is also important to reconsider how these aspects of Self manage and function within our present respective environments.

In closing, there is a simplicity and serenity that I have experienced in life while observing animals especially and humans occasionally. Somehow the traits that define our collective human environment have changed and intensified its direction away from simplicity and serenity. Presently, the focuses that dominate and take precedence within our cultures are the intense, high adrenaline and stress causing competitive traits. These traits are reinforced by our profound and questionable addiction to *drama* and our various ways of being *entertained*. Our differences are amplified and exaggerated and dominate our thinking and actions. We have lost and are unaware of the traits we share in common. We collectively have no tolerance and have lost our civility, integrity and sense of right and wrong. Instead power is admired regardless of how it was or is achieved. Conflict and war is promoted and so is the control of others. The others are stripped of their sense of self and systematically bound and dependent; physically, mentally, emotionally and or spiritually. There are no exceptions and no accidents; it was created this way by design and rule. These actions directly undermine, prohibit and restrict our experiences of serenity and simplicity, that are the basic needs and rights of all beings.

... So for now I ask you to stop for a moment, breathe, consider and imagine... the magic of a flock of birds flying and moving as one... a school of fish swimming and moving as one.... a herd of horses in an open field galloping as one... a pod of dolphins leaping and playing in the water as one. They move as one, no one is left out, no one is abandoned...and when they stop to eat and drink, rest and groom, play, work or just be; each is their individual self, being with each other. This analogy is worth mentioning because many of our collective illnesses are created and perpetuated by our collective cultural environments, where many are abandoned and left out. Perhaps we should follow the ways of our fellow creatures and stop the vicious cycle that each person is empowered to minimize. Collectively we minimize exclusion by taking responsibility for our personal evolution, which will always lead to inclusion.

This book comes equipped with a potential box of tools. Each tool can do something: extract a bad habit, adjust or tweak an emotion that no longer serves, hammer out alternative ideas and embody those that resonate with you. In other words, choose to authentically fix those flaws that are revealed that block or diminish or lack consciousness of Self. Through our own efforts to become more conscious, we begin to identify those parts of us that get in the way, that prevent the emerging consciousness from manifesting. As we resolve those aspects that got in the way, we reconnect the mind and the heart with spirit. Allowing the Self to emerge is purely based on our ability to become more and more conscious. Our divinity is already there; we bring it forth by unblocking, clearing a path and allowing higher consciousness to surface and manifest in our lives first. As more of us become more conscious, the corresponding reflection will become more and more evident in our world. A more conscious world is and will and can only BE through our own efforts. There is no other way.

Part 1 Sacred Geometry Basics
How it relates to life and the Human Body

Phi Ratio: The Blueprint of Life (One Dimensional Line)
Fibonacci Sequence
Fibonacci or Golden Spiral (Three Dimensional Plane)
Golden Means Rectangle (Two Dimensional Plane)
PHI Ratio of the Human Body
Creation Manifests:
    1. First 7 days: Genesis
    2. Egg of Life, Seed of Life and the Fruit of Life
    3. Flower of Life
Creation Continues to Manifest: the Elements
    1. Metatron's Cube
    2. Platonic Solids
    3. Pillars of Life
Universal Language Math and Geometry
DNA, Health and Epigenetics

PHI Ratio, the "Blueprint" of Life

The One Dimensional Line

When we talk about the human body, the animal body or even the structure of all plants and ANYTHING that has life in it, without talking about their relationship to PHI, we are leaving out one of the most important aspects of what we all share. PHI, throughout history, has been referred in these various terms: divine or golden ratio, the golden mean rectangle, divine proportion or cut, or golden section. PHI is purely mathematical and is the base of geometrical forms. PHI is actually a "blueprint" of everything in nature, in the macro and micro worlds of life. Anyone, not just a mathematician, can understand and visually experience the wonder of PHI. Many great architects and artists have used it in their works! PHI relationships even show up in the orbits of the planets, especially between Earth and Venus and between Jupiter and Saturn. The orbits of these two sets of planets form beautiful geometric patterns based on PHI. The simple beauty of PHI is that it's just a simple line divided in exactly the right place. The structures of the human body, elephant, whale, cat, frog, plants and trees ALL have the PHI ratio used in the design of their respective forms! All of nature is in direct proportion to itself and to everything else, and the base is PHI. The same math scale (PHI) is used, but arranged or patterned differently dependent on the structure of the form. This one line below is the Divine Line and we will discover, together, the other ways it is used.

.618 .382 1

Fibonacci Sequence (is PHI based)

Fibonacci sequence is a sequence of numbers based on adding the last two numbers starting with (1 and 1= 2), so you have 1+2= 3. Then (2+3=5). Then (3+5=8). Then (5+8=13). Then (8+13= 21). Then (13+21)=34… 34+55= 89…55+89=144. Thus the Fibonacci sequence is 1,2,3,5,8,13,21,34,55,89,144…

The sequence continues in the positive direction and also in the negative direction. Fibonacci sequences are also fractals in how DNA (in the micro or negative direction) rearranges and self organizes as we become healthier. It is also how nature organizes itself when there are numerous and similar items such as seeds on a sunflower; it can arrange its seeds based on fractals of the Fibonacci sequence (see glossary in beginning of part 4 for fractal). This PHI sequence relationship is a "blueprint" that is followed in how a tree arranges its structure: trunk, main branches, branches, twigs and even leaves. It is also used in the arrangement of petals on flowers, pinecones, broccoli, seashells and many more. This sequence is used by nature to arrange or place its respective parts, which is an organized way to contribute to the total structure of its respective form.

Fibonacci was an Italian mathematician that lived around 1170. Through observation of nature he discovered this pattern and was the "first" to write it down and share it with the modern world. But history has verified that many ancient civilizations already knew about the PHI relationship. We can see evidence of it in their art and architecture (pyramids, ancient architectural sites), pottery and other artifacts.

Fibonacci Spiral is 3D vortex form of the Golden Rectangle (based on PHI).
The SQUARE portions of the rectangle below form a spiral by drawing curved lines starting from the most inner small squares (figure 1).
Start with the two single black squares (figure 1, almost center). The Fibonacci numbers are in red. (1, 1) which equals 2, following the red line from square to square (Figure 1 and 2).

    1 + 2 = 3 leads to the next square
    2 + 3 = 5 leads to the next square
    3 + 5 = 8 leads to the next square
    5 + 8 = 13 leads to the next square

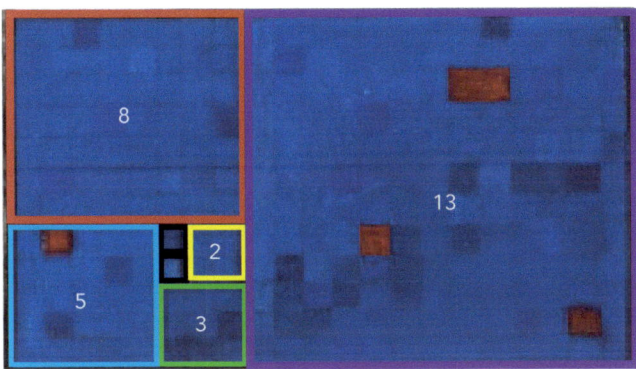

Figure 1. Golden Rectangle (2D). **Figure 2.** Fibonacci or Golden Spiral (3D).

This pattern continues by adding the last two digits in the macro world and it also continues from the 2 (1+1) black squares in the negative or micro direction (Figure 3).
Another way to see this spiral, is to start from the same place (1, 1) single black squares, curves into the yellow square box , which is 2x2 mini squares, curves into the green box of 3x3 mini squares, curves into the blue square box of 5x5 mini squares, curves into the red square box which is 8x8 mini squares and curves into the violet box that is 13x13 mini squares.

Macro and Micro Worlds
This spiral PHI pattern can also be seen in the micro world of our own DNA structure and in the macro world of seashells, the shape of a hurricane, tornadoes, and the spiral of the galaxies. See figure 3.

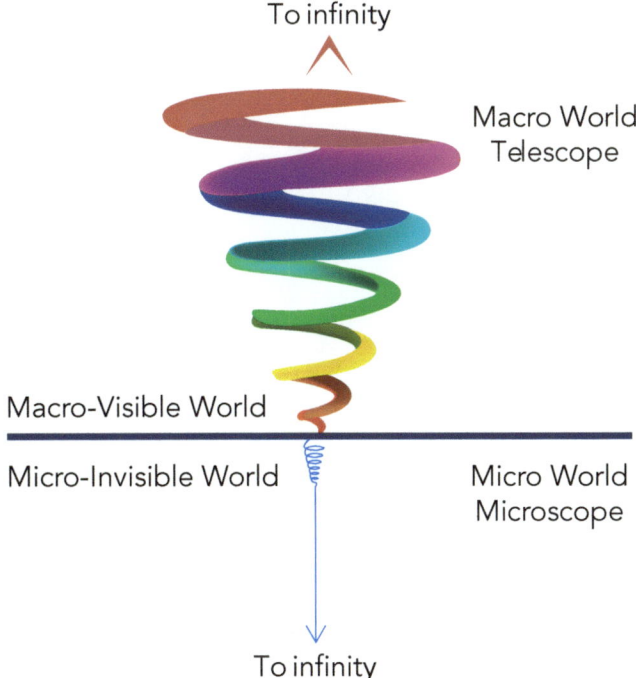

Figure 3. Side view of the Golden Spiral of the macro and micro worlds.

Golden Mean Rectangle (Two Dimensional Plane/PHI based)

If you take a square and position a compass in the middle of the bottom line of the square (see dotted slanted line, figure 3A) and proceed to draw a circle, aligning with the top corners of the square, a rectangle can be formed on each side of the square. The square plus one of the rectangles you just drew is a Golden Mean Rectangle! The other rectangle that is by itself, the violet rectangle (figure 3A) is also a Golden Mean Rectangle. When you square it (the turquoise box) in the violet Golden Mean Rectangle you get another Golden Mean Rectangle (red rectangle). This can be done to infinity in both directions, the micro and macro worlds. These PHI relations also exist in a Golden Triangle and with the Golden Pentagon (figure 4).

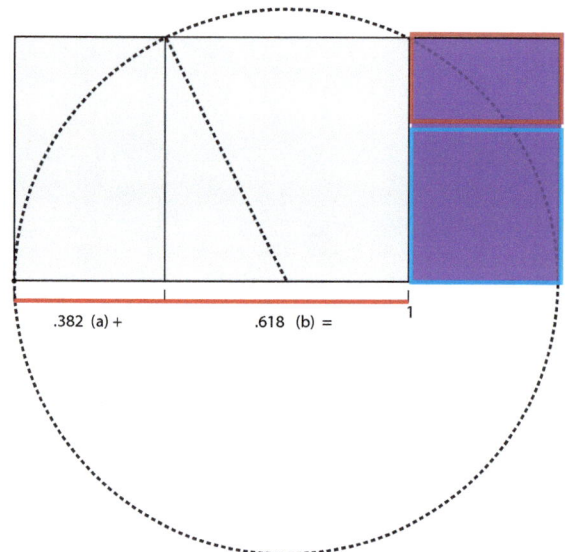
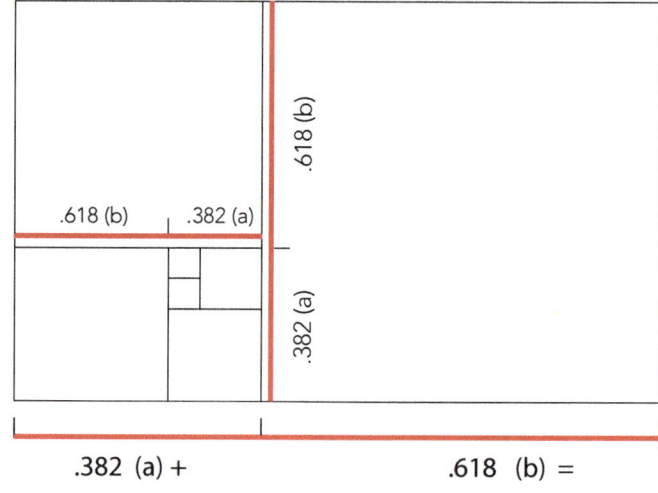

Figure 3A. How to find your own Golden Rectangle.   Figure 3B. The Golden Mean Rectangle extracted from 3A.

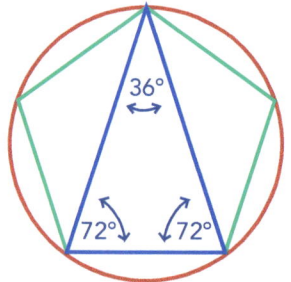
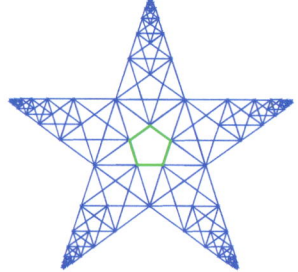
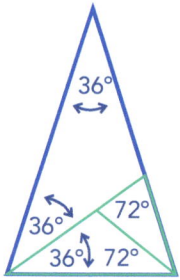

Figure 4. The Golden Pentagram and the Golden Triangle.

Many ancient as well as modern architects have used the Golden Mean Rectangle. This rectangle can be found in the architecture of many cultures all over the world, from the Egyptian pyramids to the ancient temples of Cambodia and Japan. It can also be found in the Mosques of the Middle East, the Mayan temples of Mexico, the buildings of the ancient Romans and Greeks… even the towering Gothic cathedrals of Medieval and Renaissance Europe. Today one of the most respected architects of our time was born in China. His name is Mei Pei and he is responsible for the additional structures to the Louvre Museum in Paris. He used the PHI "blueprint" in many of his works. Many artists also use this pattern as a layout in their painting compositions. Leonardo d' Vinci used it in the Last Supper, the Mona Lisa and Madonna of the Rocks, as well as other works and scientific inventions.

Divine or Golden Ratio of the Human Body Form

Divine or Golden Ratio has to do with proportions of one section being in harmony mathematically with another section of itself. We can see it everywhere because PHI is expressed in the body structures of every plant, animal and human. You can see the proportions of PHI expressed in the human body below.

Note: Divine ratios may not be in the same order for each part or portion but always use the same ratios based on PHI. Scales vary from insect size and smaller to whale size and larger and everything in between.

a. Ratio of the human body as a whole
b. Ratio of forearm, hand and fingers
c. Ratio of human DNA strand

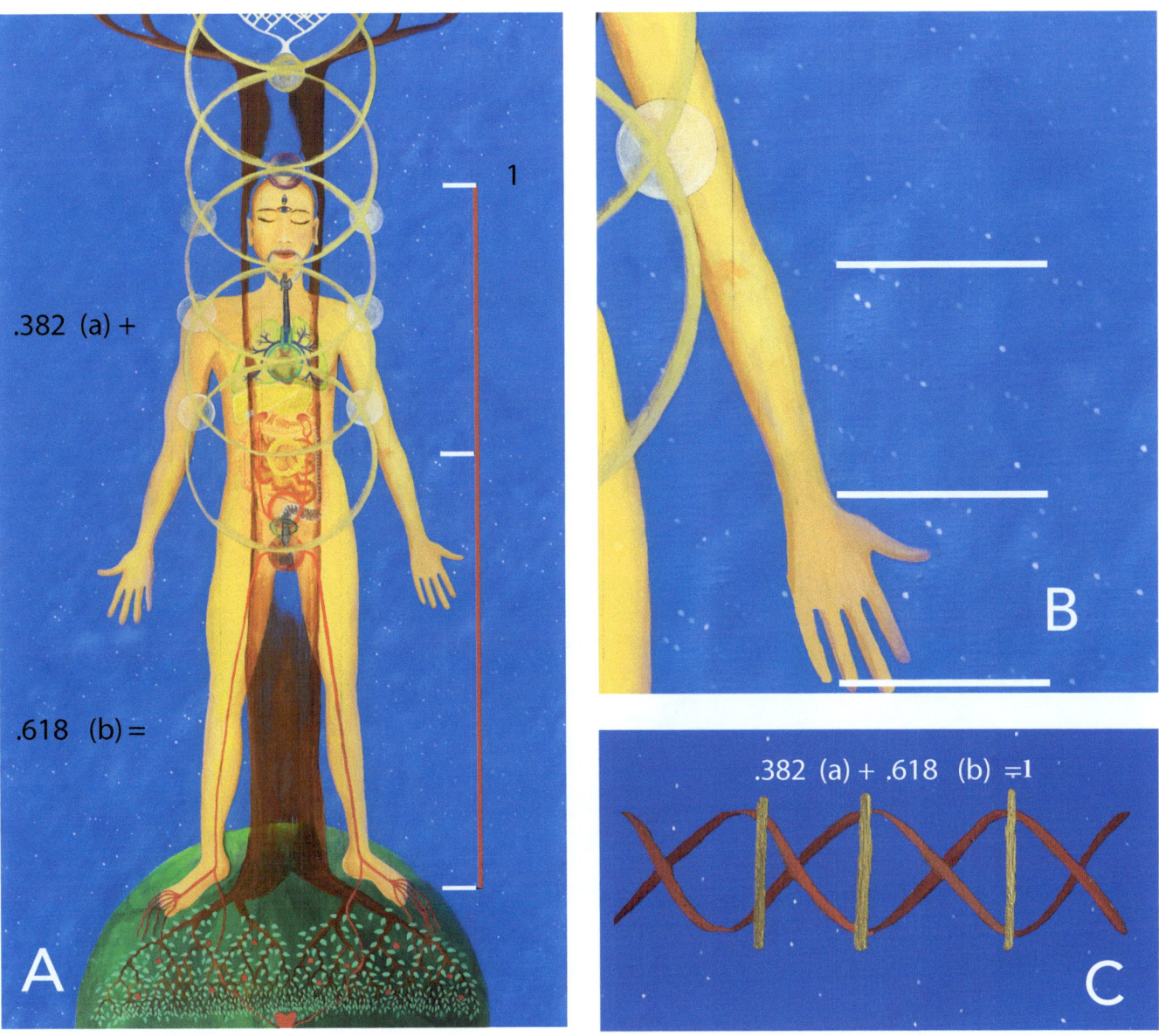

FLOWER OF LIFE, an explanation of Creation

WHERE and WHEN. The Flower of Life is one of the most ancient symbols and it is found all over the world. The world's first *recorded* civilizations, the Sumerian, Osirian and Egyptians, have this symbol written, painted and engraved on the walls of their buildings, temples and/or artifacts: bowls, plates, tablets, screens and jewelry. This symbol has been found all over the Middle East, Turkey, China, Japan, India, parts of the Americas, Scotland and France dating back to ancient times (10,000 years plus/pre-flood), as well as in medieval times.

WHAT. The Flower of Life is a symbol made up of interlocking spheres where all the spheres intersect at the radius point of each other. The first 7 spheres represent the first 7 days of creation or Genesis. This is the first stage or vortex rotation of genesis or creation.

The FIRST sphere is a spherical octahedron and it represents the CREATOR.

The second sphere, which intersects the first sphere at the radius, forms the Vescia Piscis, day one.

The third sphere joins the other 2 spheres again at the radius forming the Tripod of Life, day two.

The fourth sphere joins and intersects at the radius on day three.

The fifth sphere joins at the radius on day four.

The sixth sphere joins at the radius on day five.

The seventh sphere joins at the radius and forms the SEED of Life on day six. The Seed of Life is considered the symbol of creation and is the blueprint of the Universe. It is also the building block or starting point of Creation. Creation advances from the simple to the more complex as "spirit" or the Divine descends into matter.

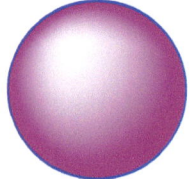

God/First Source

Spherical Octahedron. When God/Creator made or constructed our 3D world; the blueprint used is based on the sound vibrations that are based on a nine-grid system. A nine-grid system signifies that the construction of all natural forms can be numerically reduced to nine. Sound vibration is music that is in whole and half note tones. Therefore all music should be tuned to its original, consistent, harmonic and coherent frequency of 432Hz. (4+3+2=9).

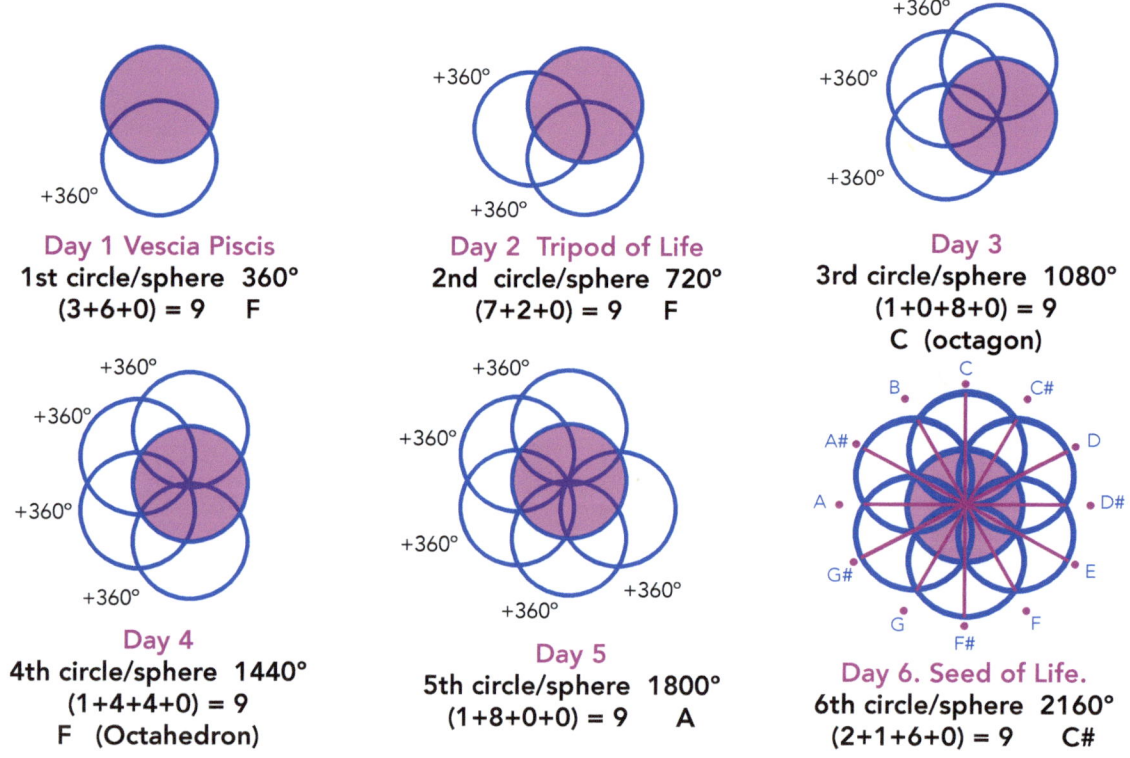

Day 1 Vescia Piscis
1st circle/sphere 360°
(3+6+0) = 9   F

Day 2 Tripod of Life
2nd circle/sphere 720°
(7+2+0) = 9   F

Day 3
3rd circle/sphere 1080°
(1+0+8+0) = 9
C (octagon)

Day 4
4th circle/sphere 1440°
(1+4+4+0) = 9
F (Octahedron)

Day 5
5th circle/sphere 1800°
(1+8+0+0) = 9   A

Day 6. Seed of Life.
6th circle/sphere 2160°
(2+1+6+0) = 9   C#

Eight spheres represent the Egg of Life and it represents the third stage of cell division in the embryo. The third stage is described as follows: first cell divides, there are then 2 cells, those 2 cells divide and they become four, those four cells divide and they become 8. Some believe that in the beginning, all life is the SAME but at the division when 4 become 8, the cells KNOW what they are or what form they will take. In other words, for the first several cell divisions an elephant, man and whale are exactly the SAME, but between the 4th and the 8th cell it becomes an elephant, or a man or a whale! The 8th sphere can also form a cube when straight lines can be drawn connecting the radius of each sphere (Figure 1). Now creation will rotate again into the next stage, the Flower of Life (Figure 2).

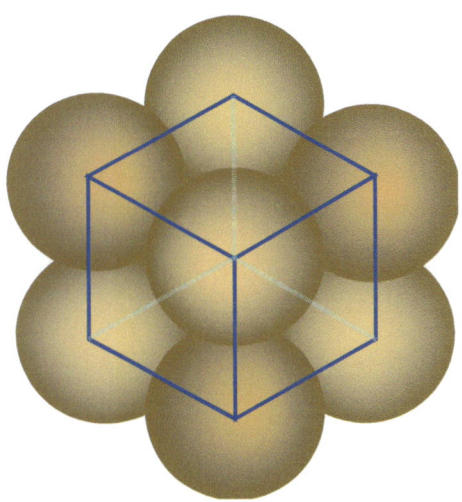

Figure 1. Egg of Life, continuation of Genesis.
First eight cells (one unseen behind forms a cube).

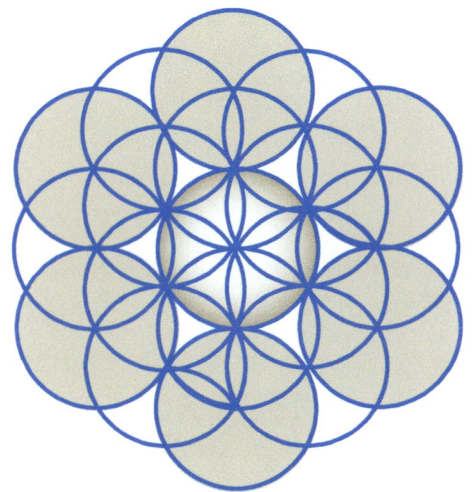

Figure 2. Flower of Life. This is the continuation of the next vortex rotation after the Egg of Life.

Nineteen spheres equals the Flower of Life. Figure 2. There are 3 spheres (circles) on the far left and right, four on the inside next to each three and five circles down the middle all interlocking at the radiuses of each other. When the spheres flatten, they become circles and this Flower of Life pattern results. As spirit descends into matter; more spheres are added during "rotations" or spinning motion. In the rotation, we evolved from the Egg of Life to the Flower of Life and now we will evolve and rotate into the Fruit of Life.

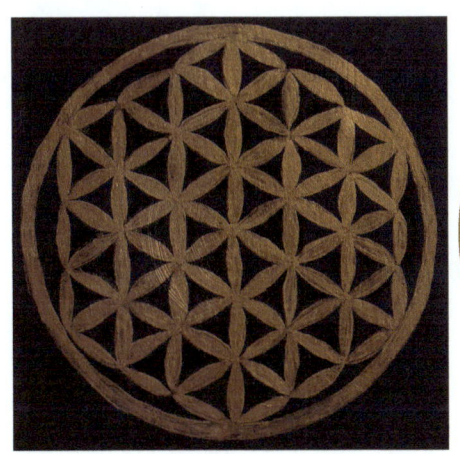 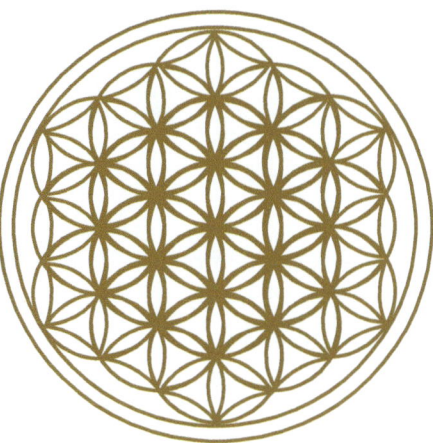 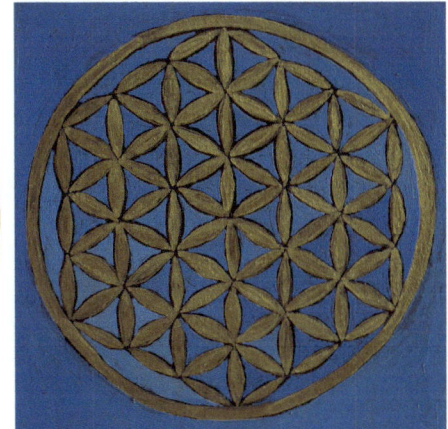

Flower of life patterns.

Fruit of Life, in 3D is 64 spheres descending into matter creating the extended version of the Flower of Life pattern, called the Fruit of Life. In the Fruit of Life there are 13 sacred spheres that help form matter, the primary elements of which our physical world manifests.

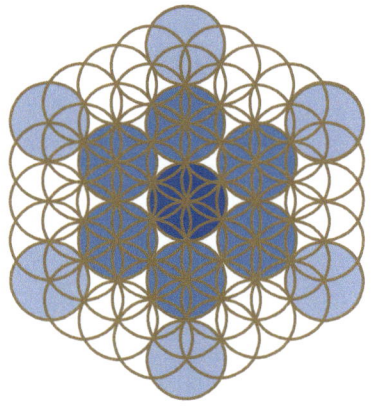

Figure 1. The Fruit of Life.

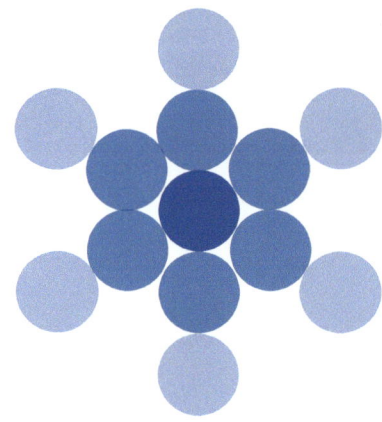

Figure 2. The 13 sacred spheres are circles extracted from The Fruit of Life.

Note. Please keep in mind the 13 sacred circles are actually suspended in 3D. There are 64 interlocking spheres of which 13 are extracted. In figure 2 the representation is in the flat 2D form.

METATRON´S CUBE and the 13 sacred spheres
Creation continues to manifest... the elements.

Within the 13 sacred spheres, lines can be drawn to form the following basic geometric shapes: the star tetrahedron, hexahedron, octahedron, dodecahedron and the icosahedron. Metatron´s Cube contains all of the geometrical forms. This is also a nine-grid system, all natural forms can be numerically reduced to nine.

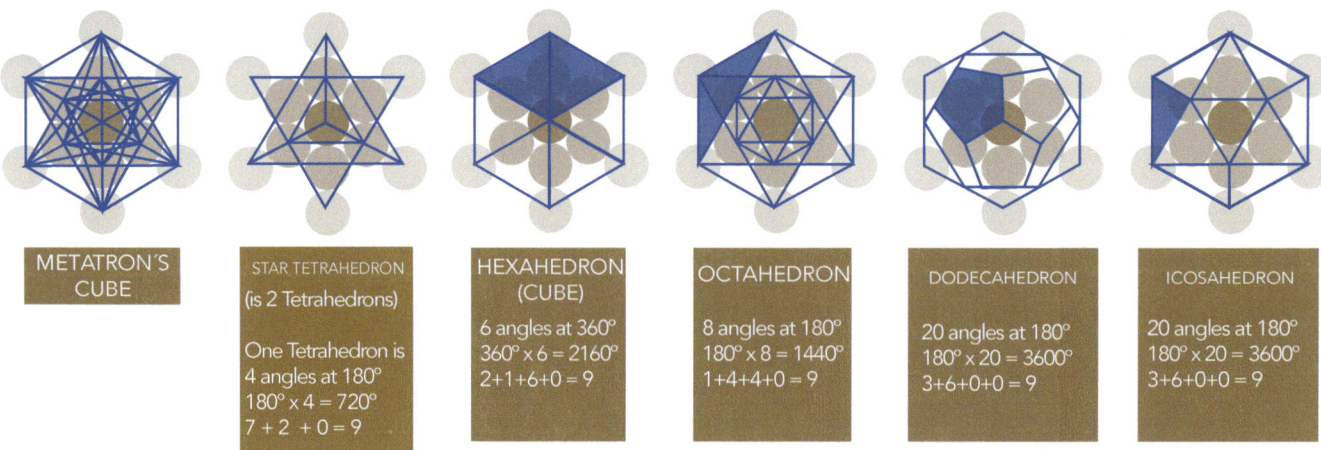

METATRON´S CUBE	STAR TETRAHEDRON (is 2 Tetrahedrons) One Tetrahedron is 4 angles at 180° 180° x 4 = 720° 7 + 2 + 0 = 9	HEXAHEDRON (CUBE) 6 angles at 360° 360° x 6 = 2160° 2+1+6+0 = 9	OCTAHEDRON 8 angles at 180° 180° x 8 = 1440° 1+4+4+0 = 9	DODECAHEDRON 20 angles at 180° 180° x 20 = 3600° 3+6+0+0 = 9	ICOSAHEDRON 20 angles at 180° 180° x 20 = 3600° 3+6+0+0 = 9

The star tetrahedron represents the element of fire and the hexahedron is the element of earth and both of these elements are considered male. The octahedron represents the element of air and the sphere represents the Void and both represent the child. The dodecahedron represents the element of ether. The icosahedron represents the element of water and both of these elements are considered feminine. All circles and spheres are considered feminine. The lines that can be drawn connecting the spheres bring matter into being (creation). The lines are considered male. **Note:** refer to Pillar of Life.

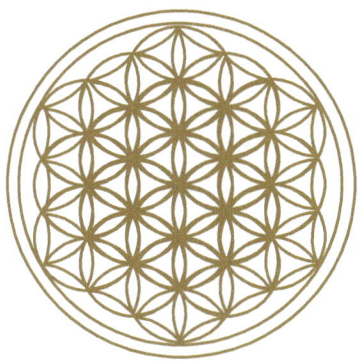 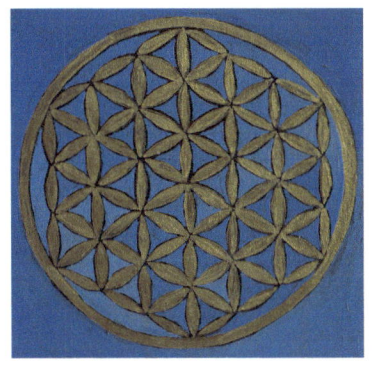 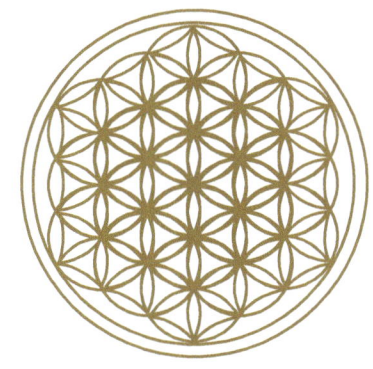

Metatron is a legendary and mythical figure. There are two different stories of who he was. Some believe he is an archangel very close to God, who came to Earth to give the people the Divine Blueprints of Creation. Others believe he was Enoch, a man from the old testament in the Christian Bible who *became* Metatron. Basically, Metatron (Enoch) is considered a scribe who took notes or lessons directly from God about the secret (blueprints) that God used for creating ITS creation. History can not trace the word "Metatron" back to any place of origin from any language on Earth.

Platonic Solids
Another explanation of creation manifesting the elements.

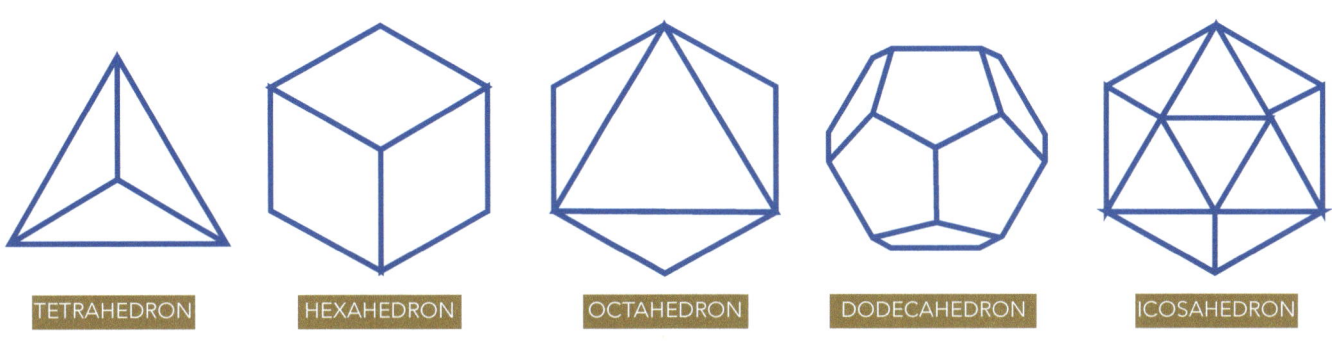

TETRAHEDRON HEXAHEDRON OCTAHEDRON DODECAHEDRON ICOSAHEDRON

The Platonic Solids are the basic geometric shapes that give form or structure to matter. They are the tetrahedron, hexahedron (cube), octahedron, dodecahedron, and the icosahedron. The differences in the Platonic Solids and Metratron's Cube is the Star Tetrahedron, which are two tetrahedrons, one tetrahedron is inverted and intersects the other tetrahedron forming a six pointed star. The other difference is Metatron realized that all these basic shapes could be formed within a cube using the 13 Sacred Spheres from the Flower of Life pattern. (See pg. 21). This links all geometric forms back to PHI, the Divine ratio.

Plato was a Greek philosopher who also taught math and geometry. He lived around 428 – 347 B.C. When he was young, he was a devoted student of Socrates. Socrates was killed for his teachings. Plato wrote down many of the teachings of Socrates in dialogue form. One of the dialogues is called "Timaeus" in which he taught that the elements came from these basic geometric forms. In time, the group of these forms were named after Plato, Platonic Solids.

Metatron's Cube, the Platonic Solids and the Three Pillars of Life
An explanation of how creation manifests and oscillates.

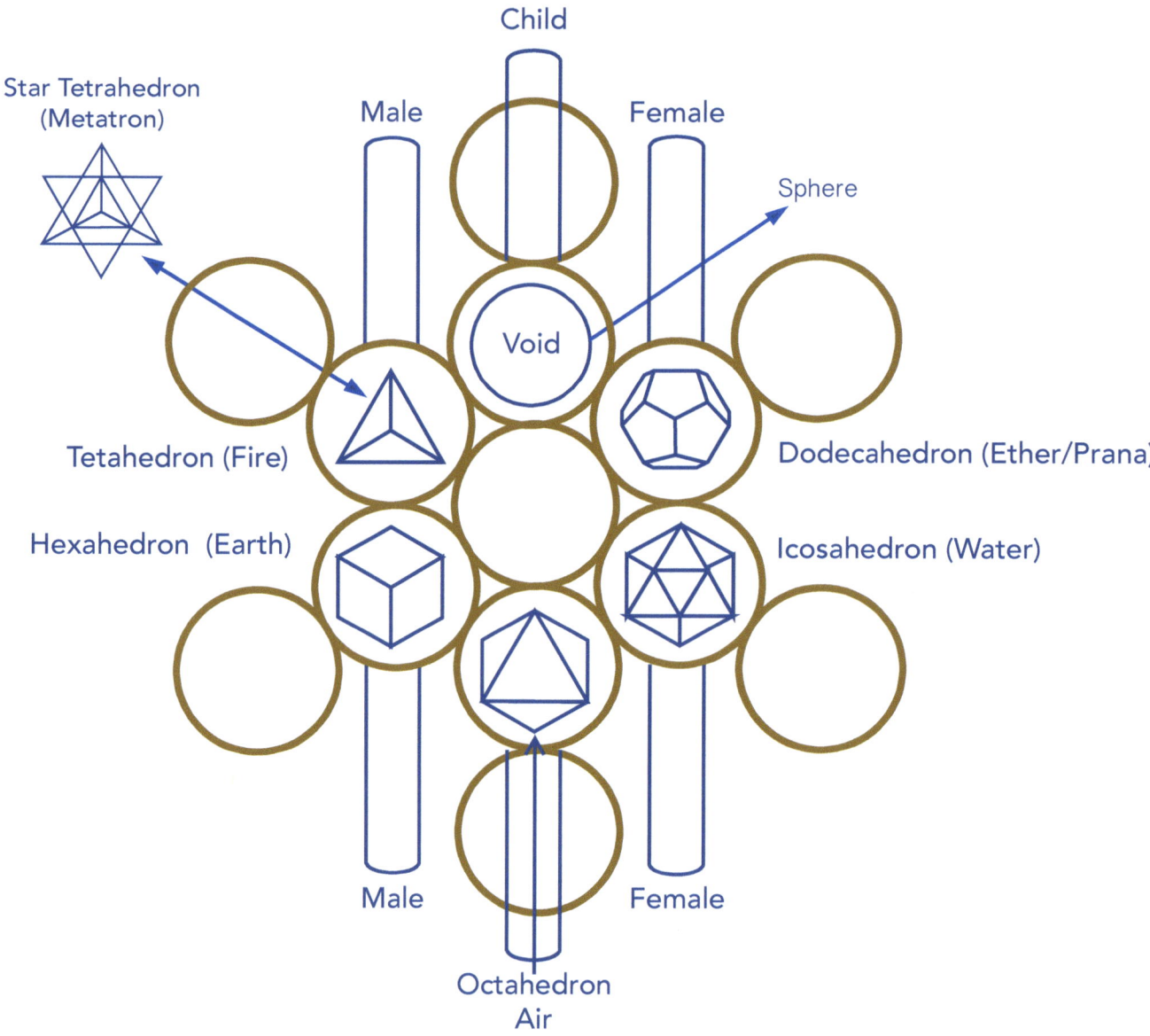

Note: The only difference in the Pillars of Life between Metatron's Cube and the Platonic Solids is the tetrahedron (Plationic Solids) and the star tetrahedron (Metatron's Cube).

The Three Pillars represent the trinity in polarity similar to the Kabbalah, discussed in Part 5. The left column represents male and left-brain and the proton of the atom. The center column represents the child and the neutron. The right column represents the female and the right side or hemisphere of the brain and the electron. The child is the link between male and female, right and left hemispheres of the brain and masculine and feminine traits. Ancient schools of wisdom believed one could connect to their higher powers and expand their consciousness when one could integrate and incorporate both male and female strengths with the innocence of a child. The nature of life will always present its wonders, as well as its challenges; the ancients realized this and found a way to live more in harmony with the duality through equanimity or balance.

The Universal Language is Math and Geometry
The Blueprint of God and why we should use these Blueprints and apply them in our lives.

Community, city and town planning, buildings, architecture, furniture, music, devices and gadgets, as well as all art forms that follow and patterns itself utilizing sacred geometry has a natural, compatible and complimentary resonance with the human body. It has this resonance because the human body, as well as all other life forms, also have their structures based on sacred geometry. This resonance of structure based on sacred geometry, creates harmony between all life forms and things (man made) and our environment.

This resonance promotes health in the body, in the mind and in the emotions and that health (anchored in equanimity) uncovers more of the untouched, non-dual, pure soul; allowing it to shine and manifest in the world. When we can establish this connected sacred geometric aspect of living, it amplifies and increases our ability to respond and interact with our self, others and the environment in a harmonious way. It also anchors the physical material world to our individual souls; this connection (or re-connection) is intelligence in motion in its highest expression.

DNA, Health and Epigenetics (Recent studies)

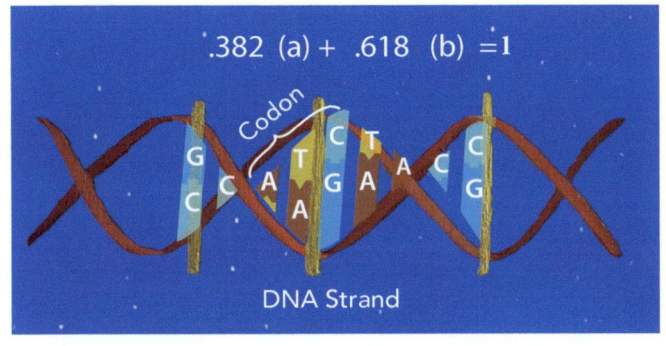

Glossary

Codon= 3 sequenced (of the four base building blocks) of DNA = encoded amino acid. There are four base or building blocks for DNA and they are nucleotides (nitrogen based): adenine (A) cytosine (C) guanine (G) and thymine (T). Any combinations of 3 sequenced nucleotide from the four base building blocks are a code for one amino acid. Amino acids are the building blocks of proteins. They (the 3 sequenced nucleotides) are a codon that can become activated (or inactivated) depending on many variables within one's own human body environment (including the ethereal bodies) and/or within one's general living environment (epigenetics). The double helix strands that hold the nucleotides are phosphates and sugar based. DNA is found in every cell of the body.

Fractals are a basic shape that is repeated over and over again. It is a self-repeating organized pattern that changes it's scale or size. Fractals exist in the microscopic world (DNA) and in macro world and beyond. A fern plant is an example: its entire structure including all the parts of its structure: the branches, leaves and veins… all share the same pattern structure, self-similar, self organized and repeated over again but on different scale.
The leaves on the tree are arranged in a fractal pattern: same shape pattern repeated over and over and changing in its scale or size.

Author's note: This is just very basic information further study is highly encouraged.

DNA and Health

Did you know that DNA structure is based on the PHI ratio and that it can self organize and can reorganize its structure based on PHI, higher frequencies and fractals? Did you also know that the more harmony, coherence and organization one has between the body, the mind and the emotions to spirit, the healthier one is? A healthier body and mind actually enables the DNA to do what it is suppose to do, which is it becomes more efficient. It can utilize ways to activate and have access to more of its parts, including the codons. The codons can become activated by the higher frequencies that we establish by making conscious choices that are beneficial to health. These choices turn the "codes" on within the DNA that allows it to improve, upgrade and/or re-organize itself based on PHI. As each DNA molecule becomes reorganized, energy flow is enhanced. The DNA can also reorganize its two meter long strand of informational codes based on the efficient fractal structure. When the DNA strand is less constricted and its components less defectively intertwined, it has improved access to more portions of itself. This is made possible by one's inspired desire to commit to making more conscious healthy life choices. These choices can actually enable the DNA, to turn on the better healthier "codes" and turn off codes that no longer serve the body, mind and/or the emotions. The 4 basic building blocks of DNA and their numerous combination possibilities plus the ability of the codons to turn on and off any of these possible sequenced combinations, is the way the body can make its own "medicine" and/or cure or remedy itself. These possibilities already exist within our DNA strand both in the known accessible portion and in the larger "no access" dormant portion, that some scientist label *junk DNA*. The liberated DNA is enabled and it can use its intelligence only when it can work in tandem with one's conscious awake Self! Our healthier diet choices and more natural calm way of truthful living raises the frequency and vibration, switching on healthier DNA codes. These higher frequencies enable the body, mind and emotions to perform as a unit at optimum levels. This activates intuition and the DNA's intelligent ability to mend and cure it self and the body, mind and emotions. It is also the ground work and foundation, which allows the already perfect soul to emerge and live in a manifested material world as a soul unit.

Step 1. Free Will - Growing desire and choosing to connect within, to Self.
A. One's spiritual efforts towards developing a more natural healthy body +
B. Developing natural healthy thoughts and calming the mind (through meditation, yoga and contemplation) +
C. Over-coming lower vibrational emotions (such as anger, greed and envy) and developing higher mature emotions such as forgiveness, kindness and empathy =
D. Balance, equanimity =
E. Coherency (between body, mind and emotions) that are established and conductive for allowing connection to one´s soul and ultimately to Spirit.

Step 2. A Coherent Self can connect and create higher frequencies= DNA activation.
a. Beneficial codes turned on and harmful codes turned off.
b. DNA becomes more organized based on PHI and
c. Constricted portions of DNA reorganizes and transforms. DNA becomes relaxed improving energy flow and re-organizes based on PHI and fractal structures.

Step 1 and 2 work in tandem with each other:
Step 1 reinforces 2 and
Step 2 reinforces 1…creating an electrical circular charge of self-mastery and self-evolution.

SeeMore and Matisse SAY...

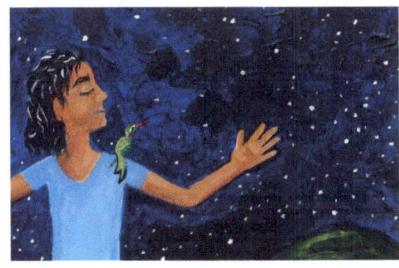

Matisse: "I don't understand exactly what this means SeeMore. It seems complicated about the DNA."
SeeMore: "Well let's explain it another way. Remember that tremor that made a mess of the hardware store?"
Matisse: "Yes!"
SeeMore: "Remember how we all went to the store to find tools but we could not find the exact tool we were looking for because everything was so disorganized?"
Matisse: "Yes…"
SeeMore: "Then remember how your uncle suggested that we should organize all the tools first: the screws, nails, power tools, hand tools, garden tools, plumbing and the electrical supplies were to be all separated and organized?"
Matisse: "Yes, yes, yes…I remember that's because I helped!"
SeeMore: " Well organizing the hardware store is like organizing your Self."
Matisse: "WHAT?"
SeeMore: "Think about it…replace everyone organizing the hardware store with YOU organizing your self: eating better foods, exercising, meditating and calming your mind…working on and eliminating your lower emotions like anger, jealousy or greed, those emotions that cause shallow breathing that tense and constrict the muscles and organs.
As the store became organized, one had more access to the tools and could use them as needed. Same is true for you as you clean up the body, mind and emotions and relax the muscles and organs; one breathes deeper, creating conditions where energy flow opens and allows for everything to work better together. This harmony (organizing) that one creates within and between different parts of the body, mind and emotions; creates a higher frequency that connects to spirit and intuition. All the effort everyone put into repairing the store: the organization of the tools, the cleaning, the assessment of damaged and useable goods, these are some of the steps that business people use to better their businesses. But what do we do to that enables our bodies, minds and emotions to work and function better as a unit?"
Matisse: "WOW! I get it now…so if I organize me and take care of me like Uncle takes care of that hardware store, then I will have a better functioning body, mind and emotions? What are the tools that will help me take better care of my body?…that will help me calm my mind?…and what will help me lower or get rid of constricting emotions like anger, greed and jealousy? And by doing all this, will the tools help me with my… life?!"
SeeMore: "YES, big yes and this book is a way to discover some of those tools that will help us heal and connect the body, mind and emotions to spirit. These tools will lead us towards activating the most important aspect of our human body…"
Matisse: "Does it have to do with DNA?"
SeeMore: "When you do all these things to help yourself heal…its activates something within you and that something will also help you, help YOU…"
Matisse: "I know, I know, it's the DNA!!!!! So when I make the choice to make better choices for my body, my mind and my emotions and they are working in harmony together, that harmony creates and activates better health so that is step 1? I remember learning and experiencing some of this when I accidentally learned how to meditate (in book one)."
SeeMore: "Yes Matisse and better health connects with spirit and to your soul: its the part of who we truly are, that naturally leads to a DNA activation process …step 2. Step 1 and 2, work in tandem. When we make choices that elevate and enhance our health, we increase the probability of reorganizing portions of our own DNA including codons. We also increase our mental capacities and our emotions mature and become more stable. This creates the perfect *atmosphere* for the soul to emerge and BE."
Matisse: "WOW, this is truly magical."

Part 2 Glands of the Endocrine System of the Human Body

Adrenal Glands
Gonads Glands (male and female)
Pancreas Gland
Thymus Gland
Thyroid Gland
Parathyroid Glands
Hypothalamus Gland
Pituitary Gland
Pineal Gland

GLOSSARY for use with Glands

Organism is an individual life form such as plants, animals, insects, and fungus. Some life-forms have highly organized systems that are made up of interdependent parts that are contained in a body. These life forms: can react to stimuli, reproduce, grow, digest etc. and maintain a balance within their own individual body. Some organisms have very complex systems like humans, dolphins, elephants and whales.

Chakra and Yoga. Chakra is from the Sanskrit word "cakra" meaning wheel or circle. The full Eastern meaning and its connections are explored here; in the West its significance has been greatly reduced. In the East, chakra is a term used in conjunction with the word Yoga that means union. Union refers to the cohesion between body, mind, emotions and actions connecting them to one's soul; this cohesion evolves into realization that connects you to God/First Source and all of creation.

Chakra. There are seven centers of consciousness that begin at the base of the spine and travel up to the brain. At each center there is a concentration of energy, a hub that radiates rays of life giving light. As each hub wheel of radiating life opens, like the petals of a lotus flower, it awakens each center as the energy continues up to awaken and open the next hub of radiating light. The more petals of the lotus flower that opens at each hub, the more the reflective radiating energy can ascend.

At the base chakra, the flower is closed and constricted, as one awakens the petals loosen, open and expand towards the light. This is a metaphor that describes what happens when one masters the lower emotions and expands up and out to higher inclusive emotions, such as compassion. The soul descended or came into matter or embodiment to experience the material world. There then comes a time when one awakens and desires to ascend out of the material world or re-unite or have union again with the Divine. Meditation is the key that unlocks each center along with rightful actions. The lotus flower will fully open in the brain in the pineal gland, the 7th major and highest chakra, only after it has ascended through and awakened the life-giving light in each of the lower six major chakras.

Different groups acknowledge only the major 7 chakras or all 13 major and minor chakras or any other given acknowledged chakras between 7 and 13. This book will address 13 chakras of embodiment with the Eastern definition of union.

The Endocrine System is a collection of glands of an organism (humans) that secrete hormones directly into the circulatory system (blood) to be carried towards targeted organs to carry out specific instructions. See examples below.

Hormones are a class of signaling molecules produced in the glands and are transported by the blood to the organs to regulate physiological functions and/or respective behaviors. Some hormones inhibit certain functions and some hormones activate certain functions. Both types of hormones are needed in regulating the body in regards to timing and specific functions.

Hormones are the messengers that signal to their respective systems and organs what to do or not to do.

Examples of the two definitions

Thyroid Gland sends a hormone into the blood, targeted for the pancreas (organ) to start producing enzymes that will help break down the food into a form that the body can use, which are proteins, carbohydrates, and fats. In the new form, the body can utilize the food and feed all the cells that your body needs to live and function.

Pituitary gland and the pineal gland send hormones into the blood signaling to the gonad glands that it is time to go from childhood into puberty. In males a transition period will begin where certain organs will develop and become more functional: sperm production, muscular development, voice changes, facial and body hair growth etc. Females will undergo a similar feminine process where certain organs will be activated: ovaries to commence menstruation, growth of mammary glands for eventual lactation, widening of hips for birthing purposes etc.

Adrenal Glands   Endocrine System   ROOT CHAKRA   Light color: Red

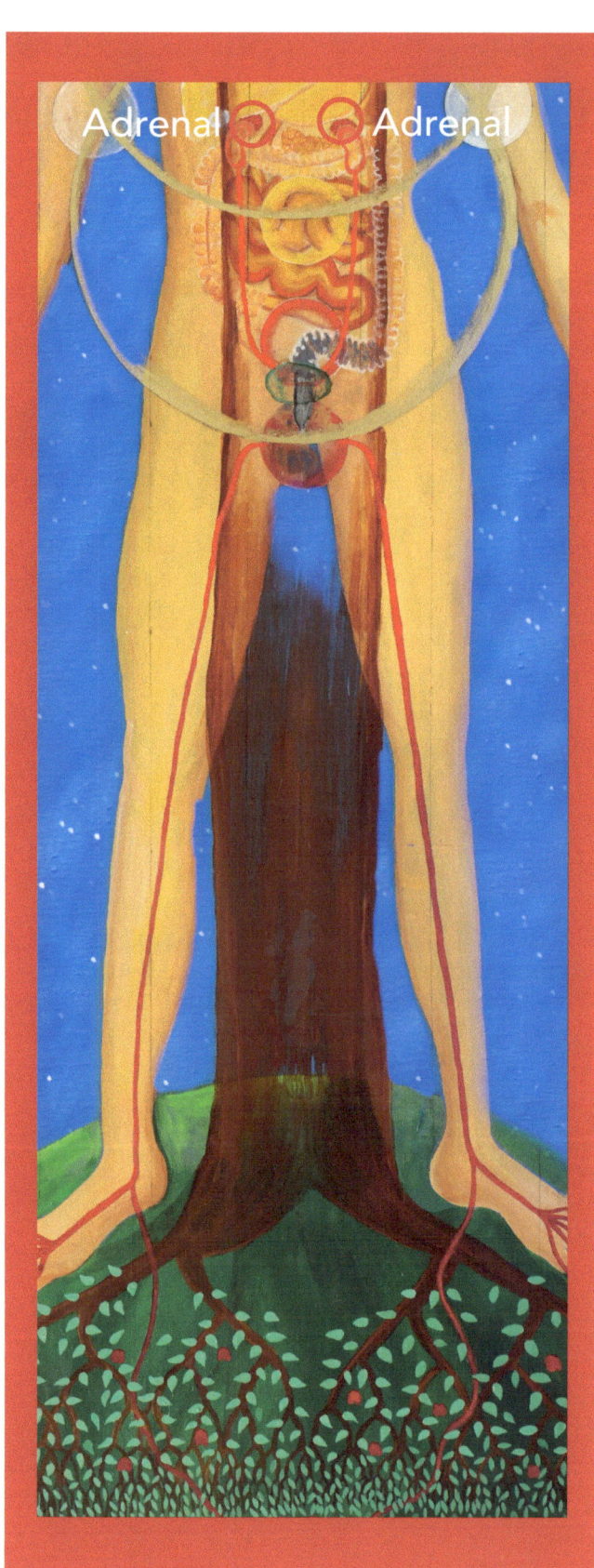

Location. The two adrenal glands are located in the lower back, sitting right on top of each kidney. They are pyramid shaped, 1.5 wide by 3 inches tall.

Function. The outside layer of the adrenal produces two main vital hormones, which are triggered by the hypothalamus gland and pituitary gland. One hormone is cortisol, it regulates how the body converts fats, proteins and carbohydrates into energy. It also regulates blood pressure and cardiovascular function. Aldosterone is the other hormone, it helps maintain the right balance of salt and water while helping to control blood pressure. The medulla, the interior portion of the adrenal, produces about another 40 hormones that help the body react to physical and mental stress such as: swelling, inflammation, allergic reactions, environmental allergens, cancer, infection, drugs and alcohol. In mid life they become a major source of sex hormones that circulate in the body to help keep it youthful. This added function happens when the gonads cease to produce sufficient hormones, usually due to the aging process. The adrenals in some way affect the functioning of every single gland, organ and tissue in the body.

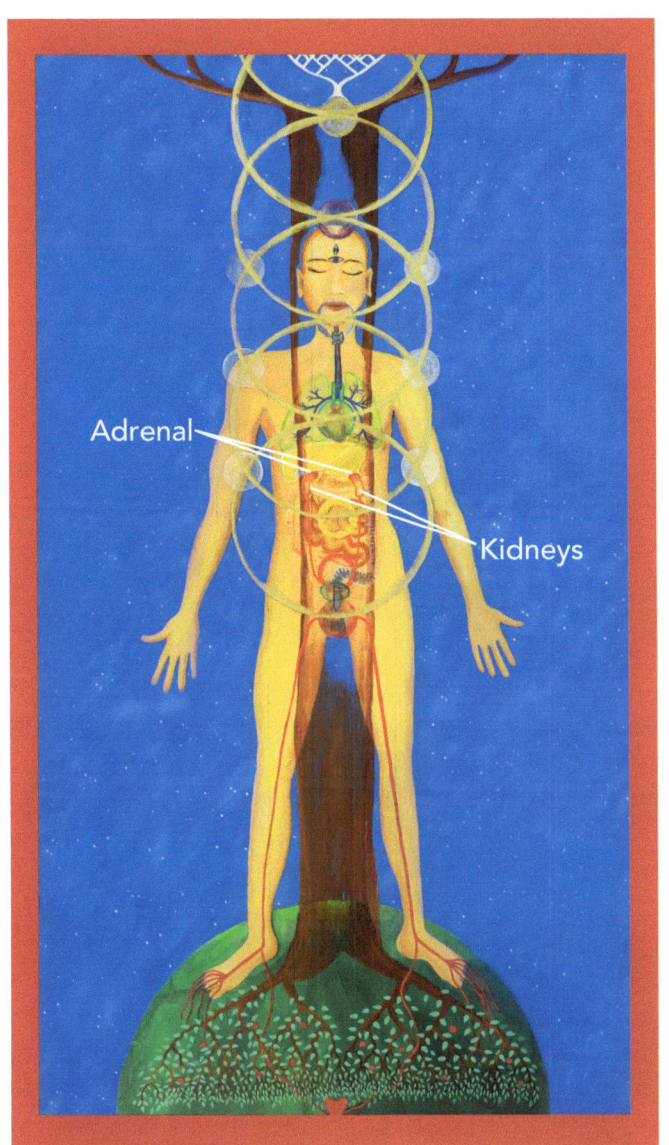

Spiritual Significance. The root chakra has to do self-preservation with being grounded and connected to Earth. The root chakra also has to do with feelings about security, safety, survival, stability, sex, fear, work and career. One's emotional feelings about the above mentioned subjects connect and permeate into the Earth.

Our "root" is the contact and manifestation chakra with Earth as a living Being. Our most basic instincts and our most high ideals and everything in between effects or causes an action or reaction that reflects our ability or lack of ability to relate to the Earth. It also affects what we manifest while on the Earth. Everything we do or don't do, everything we feel and express emanates from or has its base in either love or fear. Our connection to Earth can "ground" in the fear or the love. The responsibility is ours. When we ground love into the Earth, ALL can heal.

This is the chakra of self preservation, which includes vagina, penis, pelvis, legs, feet and tailbone.

SeeMore and Matisse say, the adrenal glands help regulate the conversion of fats, carbohydrates and proteins into energy that your body can use. This energy goes to all the other glands and organs, including your brain and heart, helping them all work well together as a unit. It is also known as the *flight or fight* gland because when we become afraid our heart beats faster and our minds are on alert while we are deciding to fight or run…it continues to give us this added energy until we feel safe. Fear over-uses the adrenals glands because it keeps us in a state of constant alert for danger. It is important to rest the adrenal glands by becoming a more peaceful person.

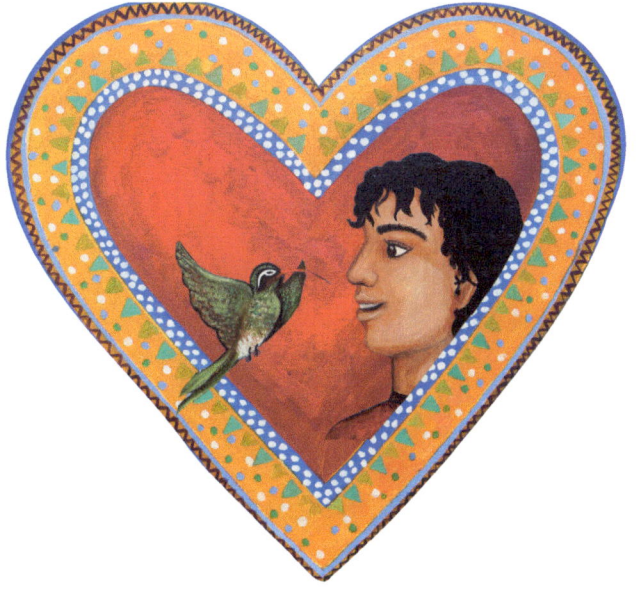

Gonad Glands   Endocrine System   SACRAL PLEXUS CHAKRA   Light color: Orange

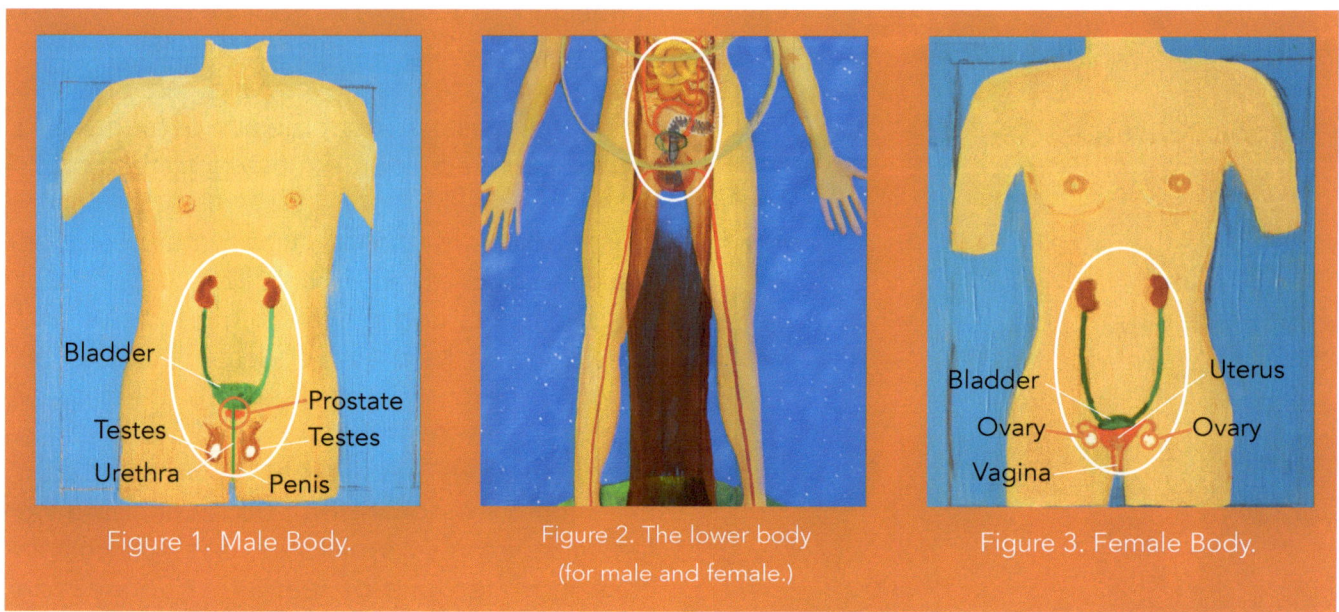

Figure 1. Male Body.

Figure 2. The lower body (for male and female.)

Figure 3. Female Body.

Location. There are two gonad glands in females called ovaries and there are two gonad glands in the male called testes. The gonads in the females are located below the navel, within the body, above the vagina. The gonads in the male are outside of the body, in the testicular sacs that are on each side of penis (see figures 1 and 3).

Function. The gonads are the physical center for reproduction cells called gametes for procreation (creating a new life), ½ from the ovaries (eggs) and ½ from the testes (sperm). The gonads control, protect and energize the eggs and sperm (respectively) and function in conjunction with the sex organs: vagina (female) and penis (male). The urethra and prostate (in males) also are part of this system. The male testes produce the hormone androgens: testosterone and inhibin (figure 1). The testicles are located in the testicular sacs located on each side of the penis it is where the sperm is produced. The testes or testicles also are where the male hormone testosterone are produced and secreted. This hormone is responsible for development of male characteristics. The female ovaries produce hormone estrogens: estradiol, progestin and inhibin (figure 3). The ovaries are located and connected on each side of the upper portion of the uterus. The ovaries are the primary reproductive organs in females and their role is connected to the male's reproductive system. The ovaries have three functions: they secrete hormones, they protect ALL the eggs that each female is born with and they release eggs (which starts in puberty) for possible fertilization. The testes are the major part in the reproductive system in the male's role (sperm) along with the female counter part, the ovaries (eggs).
Note: SeeMore and Matisse will explain this further.

Prostate Gland (male body only, Figure 1).
Location. The prostate is just below the bladder. The urethra tube starts in the bladder and travels through the prostate and the penis. The prostate is about the size and shape of a chestnut or walnut.

Function. The urethra is a transport system for the fluid that is produced in the prostate and for the sperm produced in the testes. The prostate ejects its fluid through a set of tubes and at the same time the testes release the sperm that are also ejected through another set of tubes. Both fluids meet, mix and go out through the urethra at the same time.

The prostate produces the fluid that transports and nourishes the sperm. This fluid is called seminal fluid; it mixes with the sperm that is produced in the testes. Together they travel down the same urethra tube out of the body. Only seminal fluid with sperm can pass through the urethra with an erect penis; this is called ejaculation. Urine also passes through the urethra but only when the penis is relaxed; this is called urination. The penis can only perform one function at a time, urination, ejaculation or rest.

Spiritual Significance of Gonads. The spiritual significance is to transmute, not suppress, sexual energy from lower creativity, which involves procreation or making babies into higher creativity, which involves the act of becoming more conscious that can lead to self-realization. Sexual energy can be utilized as it moves up the chakras to the higher chakras (heart and above). This movement happens as we spiritually mature by overcoming our fears and other lower emotions…the sexual energy is then transmuted and activates the higher chakras where love, kindness, intelligence, illumination and divine oneness can be expressed. This second chakra (of procreation) has a strong connection to the throat chakra, which is the center for higher creativity that includes all of the arts. This is also the chakra of self gratification, which includes the spleen, urinary and reproductive systems.

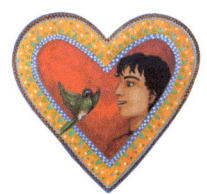

SeeMore and Matisse say, when we become adults we become capable of making babies through the act of having sex or making love. The action of making a baby is called procreation. This section of the book refers to the glands that are involved in procreation. The male gonad glands send hormonal messages to activate the male body during puberty, which is when a boy's body matures into an adult male body. Some of the hormones activated cause the following changes: sperm production, developing muscle mass, voice changes and hair growth in pubic area, face, arms, legs and chest. Hormonal messages are also sent to a girl's body; her gonad glands will send messages to her body to mature into a woman's body. Some of the hormones activated initiate: menstruation, breast growth, hair growth in the pubic area and hip carriage changes. Along with the physical changes there are also the accompanied corresponding emotional development and maturation changes for both male and female (emergence of independence, separation with parents, emergence of self reliance, etc.). In other words, when a child's body (male and female) goes through puberty (which takes several years) and their respective bodies mature sufficiently, they become capable of procreation or making a baby. This section explained what happens in relationship to the endocrine or hormonal part of a boy's body maturing (puberty) enabling him to produce sperm and the female body maturing enabling her to activate the release of eggs and what happens immediately after the egg and sperm meet, which is procreation. HOW the sperm and the egg meet through the act of making love/having sex/procreation is explained from the organ point of view in the ORGAN section of this book.

Spiritual Significance. There is another and higher type of creation that can take place when we learn to take our sexual energy and transmute it or change it into a love and kindness towards all: plants, animals, things and all other human beings. The process of this evolution eventually leads towards illumination or self-realization. We each can accomplish this by finding the "God/good" that dwells within you as You. Meditation and rightful actions help one transmute this energy. This process of transmutation eventually awakens one into a spiritual being having a human experience, rather than a human being who has occasional spiritual experiences. Spiritual experiences are feelings and BE-ing in Oneness where there are no thoughts or feelings of separation with anyone or anything. Everything is an expression of God/First Source and those expressions never repeat and are infinite in number! In part 4 and 5 we will learn ways to transmute energies from the second procreative chakra, as well as Kundalini and Chi energies, up into the higher chakras.

Pancreas Gland   Endocrine System   NAVEL/SOLAR PLEXUS CHAKRA

Light color: Yellow

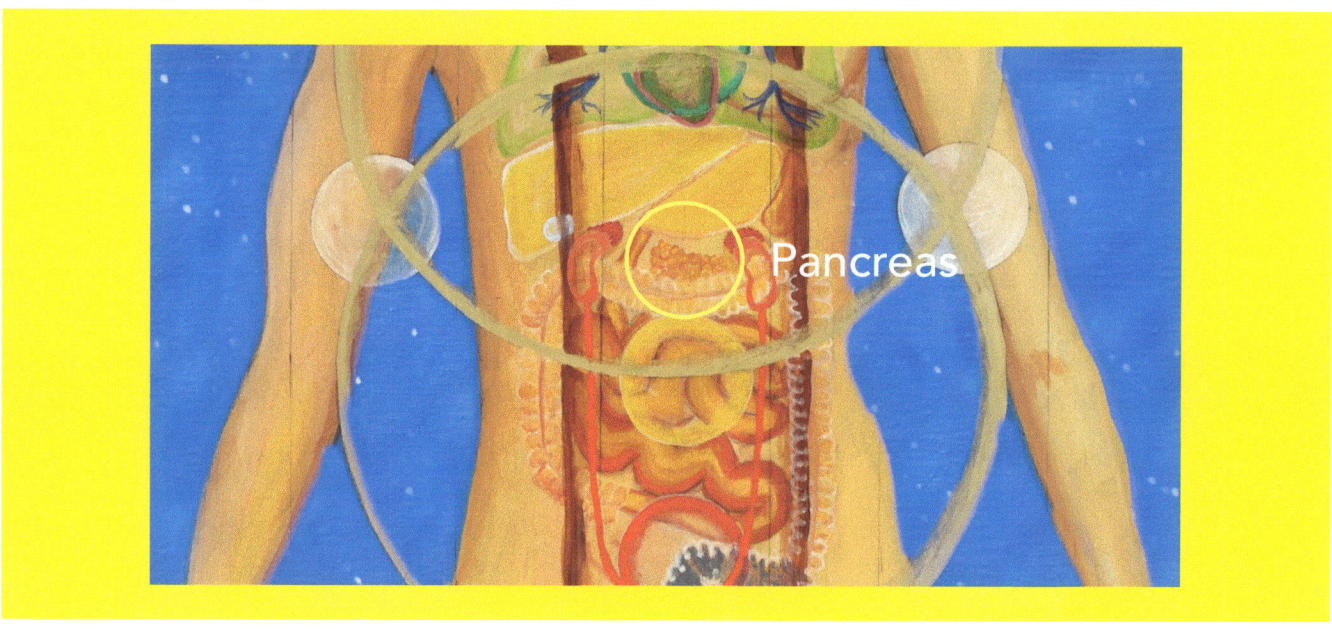

Location. The pancreas is a narrow oblong gland about 6 to 10 inches in length. It has a bumpy corn on the cob appearance. It is located in the abdomen area of the body behind the stomach. It sits horizontally across and on top of the small intestines. The head of the pancreas is connected to the entrance of small intestine by way of the pancreatic duct. Another branch of the duct also connects the pancreas to the liver and gallbladder. The pancreas secretes its own digestive juices and mixes them with the bile juices received from the gallbladder and liver and delivers them to the small intestines. All of the digestive juices will be used to break down or digest the food.

Function. The pancreas has two major functions. The exocrine (digestive) function utilizes 95% of the pancreas, producing three major digestive enzymes for breaking down fats, proteins and carbohydrates. These enzymes are deposited and stored in small ducts that lead to the central pancreatic duct ready for use in breaking down the foods and liquids that are consumed. The endocrine (hormonal) function produces two very important endocrine hormones: glucagon (alpha cells) responsible for rising blood glucose levels and insulin (beta cells), which lowers blood glucose levels. The pancreas is very important in maintaining and continuously supplying glucose, the food that feeds all cells of the body. The incorrect balance of glucose levels in the blood could cause mild to serious damage to other glands and organs. Matisse and SeeMore explain it in more detail.

Spiritual Significance. The pancreas has to do with one's energy levels: how to use one's will, how to use one's power and the availability of inner strength based on the quality of one's vitality. One can either be motivated in using these energy levels by the lower emotions or higher emotions. The pancreas is the body's battery, instinct, lower intuition and gut feeling zone.

It is the primary center for managing and overcoming lower emotions. Lower emotions include anger, hatred, prejudice, racism, envy, jealousy, lying, greed and fear. Gradual to instantaneous mastery of these emotions happens only through one's authentic development of the higher emotions. It is crucial to free oneself from the enslavement of the lower emotions. Higher emotions include: kindness, forgiveness, consideration, patience and compassion. Practice of the higher emotions, along with meditation, can dissolve and resolve the lower emotions.

The navel and solar plexus chakras are the chakra of self definition. It also includes stomach, liver, gallbladder and small intestine.

The Pancreas according to SeeMore and Matisse. When you listen to the radio, the music maybe too loud or too soft to hear. This happens because the volume isn't adjusted correctly. Well the pancreas is like the volume knob on your radio: when the glucose (blood sugar) is getting high, it sends in insulin to lower it; when the blood sugar is too low, the pancreas sends in glucose! The pituitary gland helps alert the pancreas when the "volume" or glucose portions are incorrect.

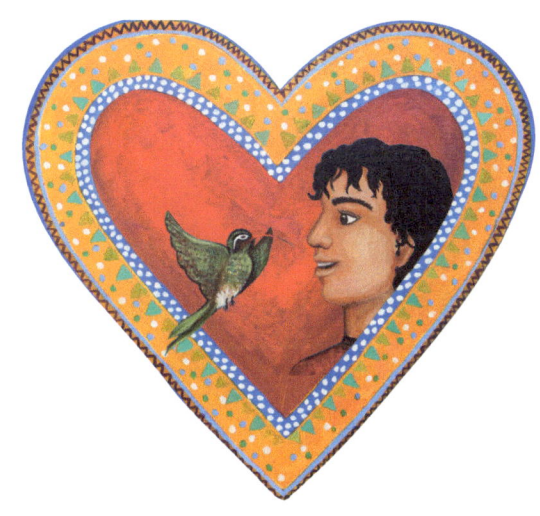

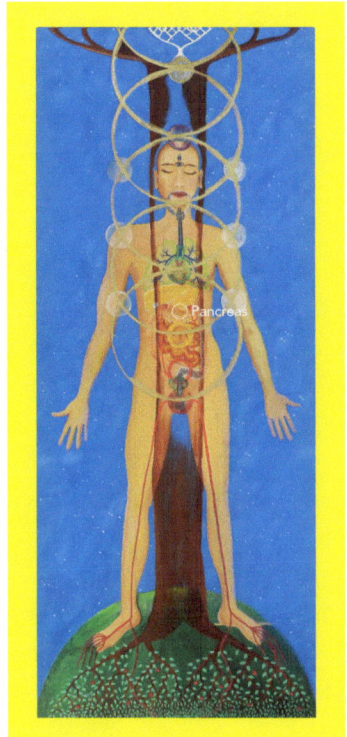

Spiritual Significance. The pancreas is also where we manage and store lower emotions, like anger. Lower emotions are powerful and destructive because they can control you rather than You controlling them. It is therefore important to resolve and transmute lower emotions like anger and fear. We can do this by taking action through meditation and by making efforts to deal with the issues that incite the lower emotions.

Note: Parts 4 and 5 discuss ways to overcome the lower emotions and how to develop the higher emotions.

Thymus Gland (Thy am us)　　Endocrine System　　HEART CHAKRA

Sometimes called the "higher heart" and "seat of intent" gland.　　Color of light: Green

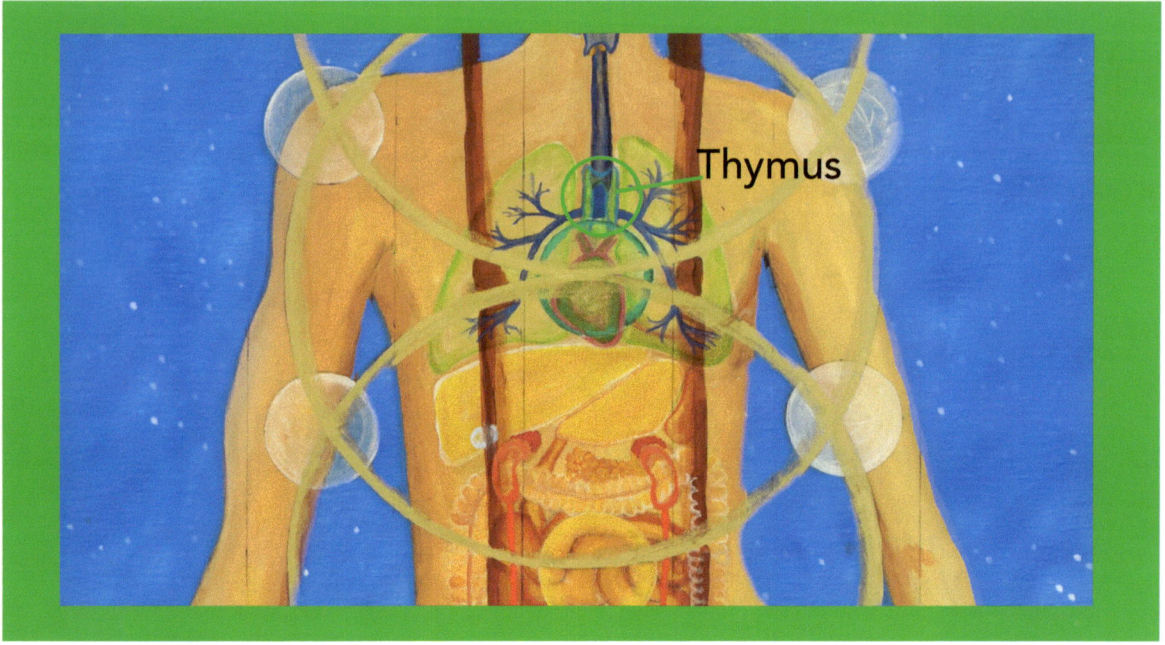

Location. The thymus gland sits on the heart, between the lungs and surrounds or wraps around the lower trachea, the tube that leads to the lungs.

Function. Thymus gland secretes hormones that enable the body to grow through the different stages of life: infancy, childhood, puberty and adulthood. It is more active in the earlier stages infancy, childhood and puberty when the immune system is developing. According to new studies after puberty it begins its decline in activity and is directly linked to the aging process, as it is less able to defend itself from diseases and illnesses.

The thymus produces the hormones that play a vital role in producing and developing the immune system's T-lymphocytes (T-cells). T-cells play a strategic role in fighting foreign pathogens (germs, bacteria and fungus) that can enter the body. There are three types of T-cells: 1) *cytotoxic T-cells* that directly terminate or kill infected cells; 2) *helper T-cells* involve the production of B-cells (that store the memory of past infections and pathogens specific to your body) and they activate other T-cells to attack the foreign invaders; and 3) *regulatory T-cells* that act as "police" to the T-cells and B-cells adding to their proficiency in protecting the body. The bone marrow is the "training area" (throughout childhood) where immature T-cells are released in the blood stream and travel to the thymus where they get further instructions. Only 2% are trained to know which cells are foreign to the body and which are not. These mature T-cells are then isolated in the cortex of the thymus until they are needed; otherwise they can have an adverse effect and become self-sensitized causing them to attack the body's own good cells. In some eastern traditions as one ages and prepares for death, emphasis is on ones spiritual evolution where universal love energy experiences are highly valued. These energies also enhance the quality of health and hence the immune system for those who connect and develop these higher subtle energy practices; especially meditation where endorphins, seratonin and melatonin are released. What better way is there but to live and leave the body with a heart full of love?

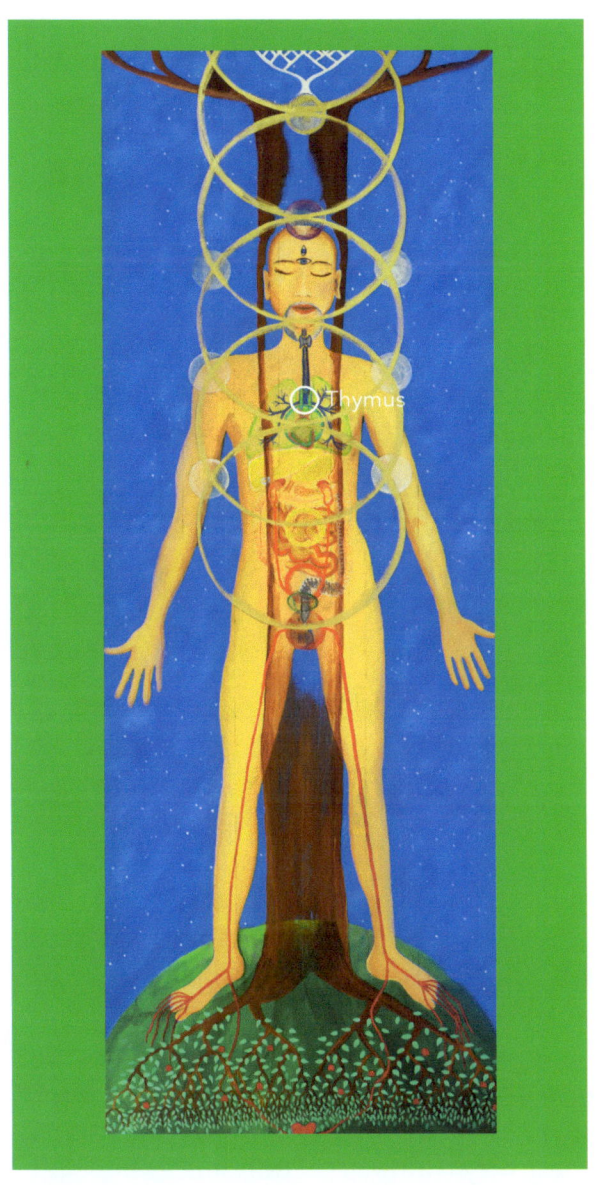

Spiritual Significance. The thymus is considered the higher heart. It connects and binds one's own heart of self love with the higher heart (thy am us) with ALL, universal love. The thymus is also closely connected and works in conjunction with the lungs (air) and throat (voice, ability to speak) and the trachea. When heart, thymus and throat are in sync or coherent, with the intent (from mind) then one experiences and lives from the higher heart. One's *seat of intent* is now working along with the heart, thymus and lungs as the intention also gets further circulated in the body via the lungs, into the blood. One's intention or motivation behind the thought is very crucial in how coherent the thymus can perform along with its allies (the heart, the throat, the lungs and the trachea).

This is the chakra of self-acceptance, and it includes lymph/immune system, blood pressure and circulation of blood.

SeeMore and Matisse say the thymus gland is shaped like a beautiful butterfly that has two long tails. The butterfly is sitting on your heart and hugs the bottom of a long pipe called the trachea. The thymus makes "soldiers": T-cells, B-cells and antigens that protect the body. They defend the body by identifying the "bad guys" like germs, bacteria and fungus that could make one sick. The thymus trains these different groups of soldiers and they all have their respective responsibilities. The most important thing to remember is that they ALL work together to make sure that the whole body is safe from germs and bacteria so the other parts of the body can do their jobs.

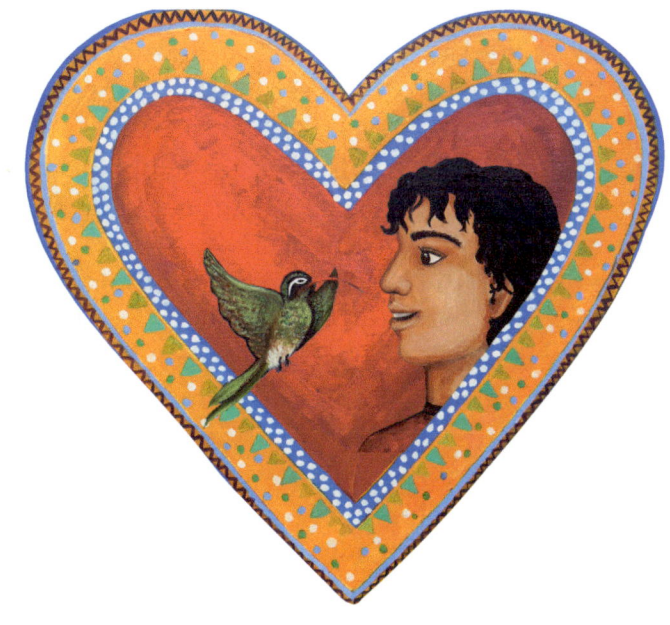

Thyroid Gland   Endocrine System   THROAT CHAKRA   Color of light: Turquoise

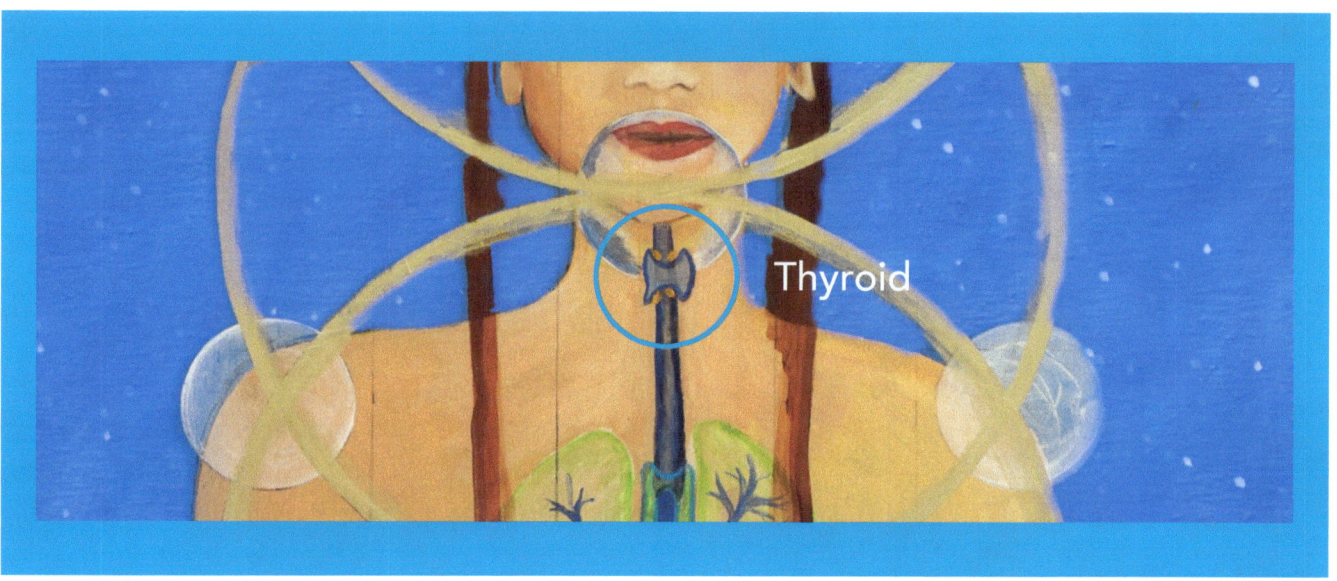

Location. The thyroid is another butterfly shaped gland located at the front base of the neck on the upper portion of the trachea. It is 2 inches long.

Function. The thyroid uses iodine taken from food to make two main hormones: Triiodothyronine (T3) and Thyroxin (T4). The thyroid works along with the hypothalamus and the pituitary glands to make sure the levels of these hormones are correct.

T3 and T4 travel throughout the body and communicate with every cell about their respective jobs. They are like the generals or boss regulators of the cells, always relaying messages about what is needed by the different parts and cells of the body. What is needed depends on what the body is doing at a particular moment. Is the body running? Then it is exercising, and will need more air from the lungs and more blood to feed all the muscle cells using the energy. Is the body eating? Then the body will need all the energy directed to the digestive organs and glands to help digest the food.

The thyroid does this by secreting hormones that control metabolism. Metabolism is how and when the body cells use energy, when the organs, glands, muscles, brain, etc. need that energy to perform certain functions, processes and activities. Some examples of how these hormones regulate vital functions as needed are: breathing, heart rate, nervous system, body weight, muscle strength, body temperature and cholesterol levels and more... these functions are affected by what the body, mind and emotions are doing and needing. Reading a book requires a different *heart rate* than when you are running. Meditating requires less energy from the *nervous system* than when you are speed racing. Different body *temperatures* are required when it is hot outside as opposed to cold and freezing. These are a few examples of the physical changes of how metabolism affects the different parts of the body when it is involved in different tasks. Metabolism also has other corresponding affects on the body: mentally (stress, worry, excessive mind chatter) and emotionally (crying/sadness, joy, anxiousness, jealousy and gratitude).

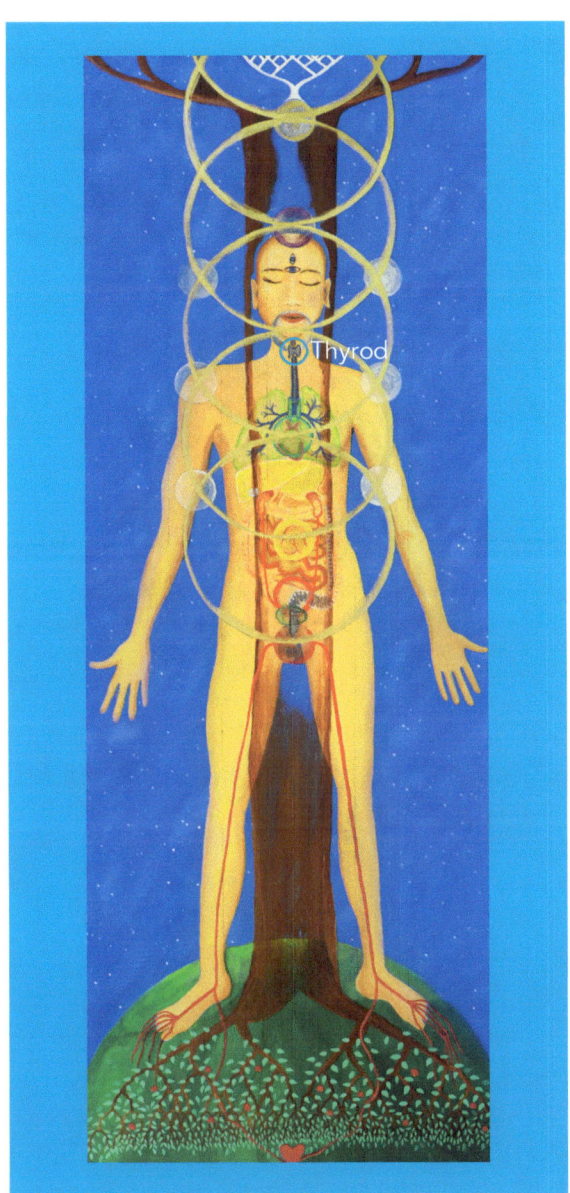

Spiritual Significance. Throat chakra deals with the ability to express, specifically with the ability to speak the truth. When one's personal truth and universal truth become ONE, then higher states of consciousness can be experienced. The original meaning of the word "kosher" meant that only pure words or truth comes out of the mouth. Truth is most important, even more important than what you put into your mouth, food.

This is also the chakra of creative expression. When the energies from the sacral procreation chakra are elevated to the throat chakra; the energy becomes transmuted into creative expressions. Creative expressions are the arts in all forms: music, literature, painting, sculpture, film, poetry, architecture, photography, graphic design, etc. The highest creative expressions are spiritual. Development of one's spiritual Self dissolves all separateness in all its forms; in thought, feeling and action. Eventually these spiritual practices lead us to ONENESS or self-realization.

This is the chakra of self expression.

SeeMore and Matisse say, that the thyroid has two generals that travel throughout the body: T3 and T4. They report to two other gland "generals," one works in the pituitary gland and the other in the hypothalamus. The goal of all the generals and their respective jobs, is the same AND are interdependent. They make sure that everything in the *engine* body with its entire cell parts (heart, lungs, stomach, etc.) are all working together correctly. They also make sure all the parts have all the energy they need to function well.

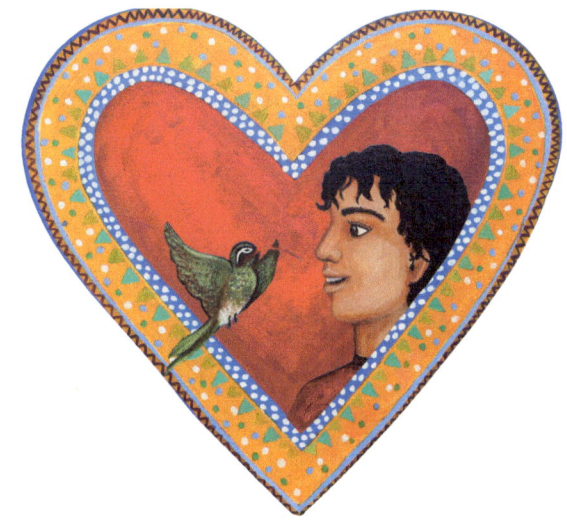

Parathyroid Gland   Endocrine System   THROAT CHAKRA   Color of light: Blue

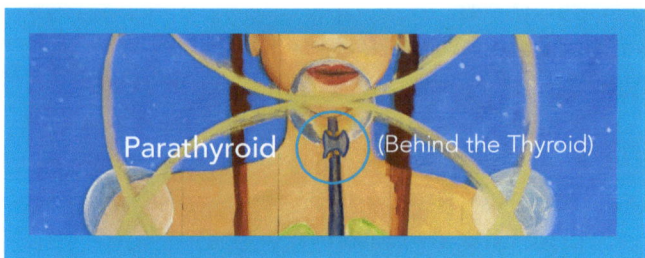

Location. The parathyroid glands are four small clusters of mini glands that are located behind the thyroid lying on the trachea.

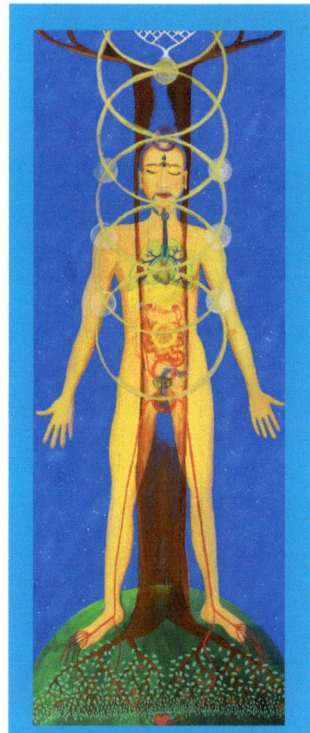

Function. The parathyroid gland secretes the parathyroid hormone (PTH). This hormone's only job is to regulate levels of calcium in the whole body. Calcium's first obligation is to the nervous system. After the needs of the nervous system have been served, the parathyroid then supplies calcium to the bones for growth and maintenance. Calcium is the only mineral that has its own gland; that's how important calcium is to your nervous system and bones. The nervous system must have sufficient amounts of calcium at all times because it facilitates the efficiency in the body's ability to communicate, which is electrical. Without the correct information communicated at the right moment, the body risks suffering from improper or crossed communication. The body communicates by sending electrical messages through the nervous system directly between the cells in a given area and from the brain to body and from body to brain. Calcium also provides electrical energy and communication to all muscles and to the skeletal system (bones).

Spiritual Significance. The parathyroid is responsible for the balancing of yin and yang. To reach truth, peace or love, a balance must be reached between the dual properties of life. Example: All beings have male and female traits within them: male is the faculty to reason, being of the mind and female represents the faculty of feelings, of the heart and emotions. Truth occurs when the male and female traits, subside and re-emerge. The alignment of the traits allows support (rather than opposition) and the *best of both* creates the balance: the balance of mind and heart. The balancing, reassessment and realignment of all dualistic traits creates more opportunities for the higher truth and hence more experiences of love and peace. This is the chakra of self expression.

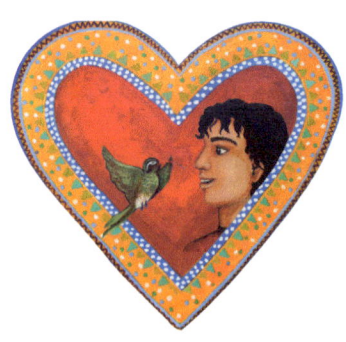

SeeMore and Matisse say, that the parathyroid takes care of ONLY one thing, calcium. Calcium is a mineral found in seafood, dairy products and some vegetables. Calcium is needed mostly by the nervous system so it can send the *radio* electrical messages correctly back and forth between the body and the brain, and directly within a given area. It is also needed for the muscles to communicate electrically, telling which muscles to use at different times: for digesting food, for resting, running, painting and fishing. Lastly, calcium is used for all the bones: for growth, for maintenance and for strengthening. The parathyroid makes sure that these different parts of your body get the right amount of calcium as it is needed.

Hypothalamus Gland   Endocrine System   THIRD EYE CHAKRA (horizontal)
Color of light: Indigo Blue

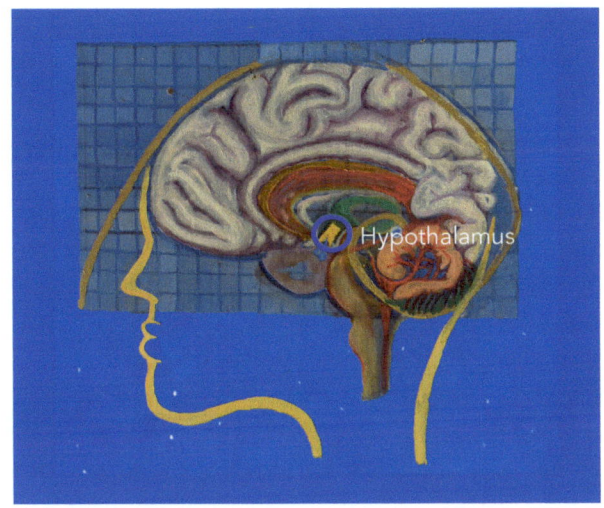

Location. The hypothalamus is located in the brain below the thalamus and above the pituitary gland and it is the size of an almond.

Function. The hypothalamus produces releasing and inhibiting hormones that work intimately with the pituitary or master gland. They work together and tell the other glands in your body to make hormones that affect and protect your health. The hypothalamus (along with the pituitary) is involved in the mediation of the entire endocrine system, as well as the automatic and behavioral functions. It does this by controlling the release of 8 major hormones that have to do with the following: temperature regulation, which

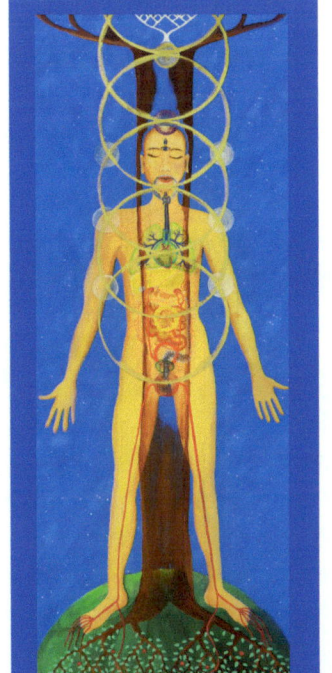

sends messages of hot and cold with corresponding behaviors sweating and shivering. It controls the food and water intake, which send messages of hunger, loss of appetite and thirst, etc. The hypothalamus also affects digestion, via the pancreas gland, sexual behavior and reproduction, via the gonad glands i.e. in puberty. It controls the daily cycles in physiological and behavioral states such as day and night/sleep and awake states. The hypothalamus moderates emotional responses via the adrenal glands: pleasure, fear, love, anger and compassion etc, with the corresponding bodily responses.

Spiritual Significance. The hypothalamus is the center of higher mental faculties and higher will. It is directly connected to solar plexus and lower will. The hypothalamus involves the ability to understand abstract concepts. It is the center of active intelligence that is inspired by the divine or self-less will. The hypothalamus gland stimulates and increases the ability for clairvoyant (hearing) experiences as well as intuitive (seeing) experiences. The hypothalamus, pituitary and pineal (inner eye, single eye) glands work together, increasing one's mental and spiritual capacities. As one develops, the inner connection between these three glands become more coherent and work in sync, which guarantees higher experiences of clairvoyance and intuition.
This is the chakra of self expression.

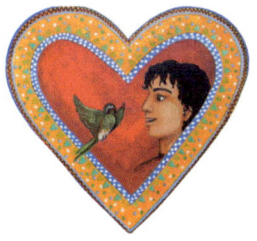

SeeMore and Matisse say that the hypothalamus gland is like a conductor in an orchestra. This gland also works with two other glands, the pituitary and the pineal. The better the glands can work together, the better the function and health of the body, mind and emotions, which promotes and accelerate the Soul's emergence. This gland is most concerned with the parts of the *orchestra* that involve the whole endocrine system, especially the adrenals, the gonads, digestive system and the regulation of body temperature.

Pituitary Gland   Endocrine System   THIRD EYE CHAKRA (horizontal)
Color of light: Indigo Blue

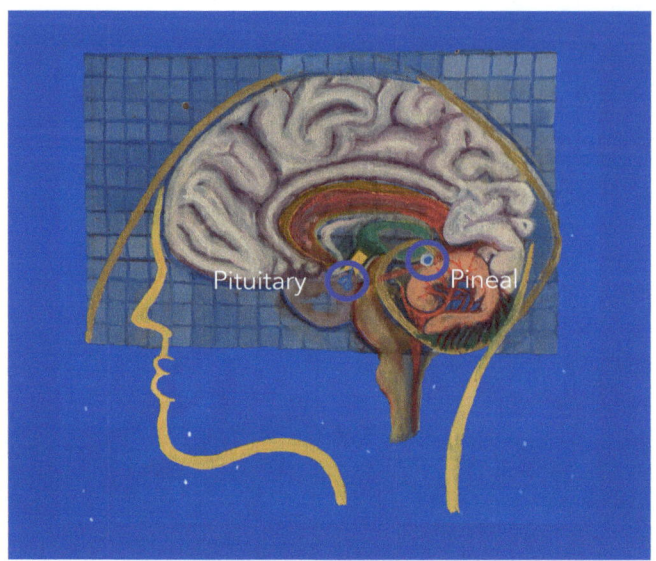

Location. The pituitary gland is the size of a pea. It is attached by a thin stalk to the base of the brain, behind the bridge of the nose. The pituitary has two distinct sides or lobes, the anterior and the posterior.

Function. The pituitary is the master gland because it controls other hormonal endocrine glands. The pituitary has anterior and posterior lobes, each with different functions. The posterior lobe does not produce hormones but is a storage place for hormones. It only secretes 2 hormones, an antidiuretic (ADH) that regulates water levels and blood pressure. The other hormones are oxytocin (in females) for uterine contraction and for lactation and testosterone (in men) for development of male reproductive tissues in the testes and prostate. The anterior lobe produces hormones of its own that are proteins and glycoproteins that are secreted and help regulate: (1) the adrenals gland for growth hormones, (2) thyroid gland and its stimulating hormones (TSH), (3) the gonad glands: ovary hormone prolactin (GH) in females and testicular hormones in males and (4) follicle stimulating hormone (FSH) for healthy skin. The pituitary also works along with the hypothalamus to determine exact needs of body for the above-mentioned glands. Another very important hormone produced in the pituitary is endorphins. Endorphins provide the "happiness" secretion for the brain and immune system in general. Endorphins contribute to the overall ease and coordination with every system within the body and their respective organs.

Spiritual Significance. The pituitary gland is also the center for psychic and higher intuition, knowing through divine perception, which is direct knowing beyond duality. Inner perception is gained through the development of intuition/Divine perception. The pituitary is also the center for higher will. Higher will is universal and is connected to lower self-will of the solar plexus. When there is a relationship between the third eye chakra and solar plexus, which involves intelligent control and discipline; evolution of the emotions, especially for understanding and compassion are inevitable. Pituitary controls left brain (rational brain), right eye, right ear and right side of the body. The pituitary is master gland because it facilitates the flow of electrical current to all other parts of the body insuring a harmony or "happiness" between all systems. Detailed information is included in part 5. This is the chakra of self-reflection.

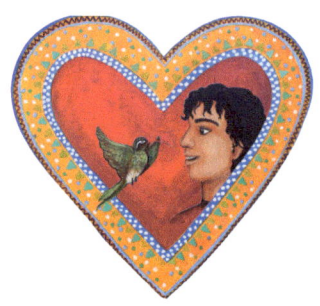

SeeMore and Matisse say. The pituitary gland is the master gland of the body. The pituitary works very closely with the hypothalamus on some glands specifically and all of the glands in general. It does this by making sure all the parts of the body have electrical currents flowing everywhere in a harmonious way. It also creates important hormones for the brain and skin. The pituitary gland is like a big conductor telling which instruments (glands) to play next, which to rest, which to play together and when all need to be playing or all resting. The "playing" or "resting" is when to turn on (releasing hormones) or off (inhibiting) hormones from their respective gland (instruments).

Pineal Gland   Endocrine System   THIRD EYE (vertical) AND CROWN CHAKRA
Color of light: Violet

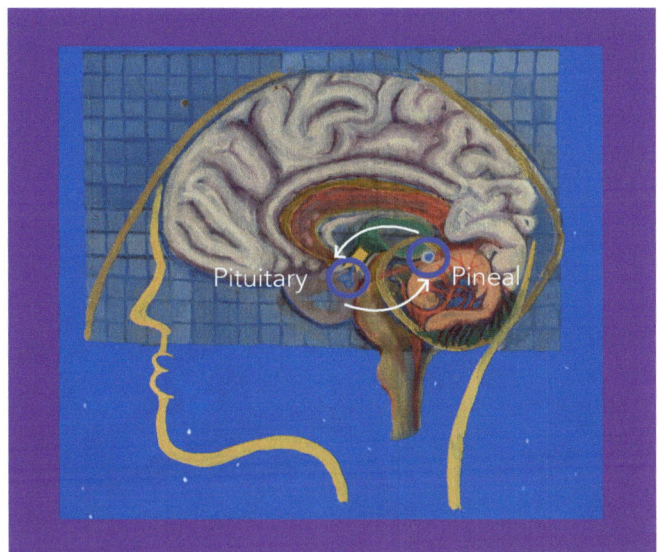

The electrical charge between the pituitary and pineal glands' (established during meditation) opens both third eyes (one is between the eyes and the other is in the center of the forehead.)

Location. The pineal gland is tucked in the groove where the 2 hemispheres of the brain come together where the thalamus is joined. It is pea size (about 8 mm) and has the shape of a pinecone. In many cultures the pinecone represents the pineal gland.

Function. The pineal gland produces and releases only one known hormone, melatonin. Melatonin affects sleep/wake patterns called circadian rhythm, it is based on 24 hour biological cycle. The pineal gland also affects the longer seasonal rhythm patterns and lifetime growth rhythms. The hormone is sensitive to light because of pineal's optical cells are sensitive to light. Light exposure lowers the secretion and darkness increases it. It also has control over the gonad glands as to the timing of puberty and aids in the proper development and functioning of respective male and female glands and organs. Melatonin is also responsible for fighting free radicals. Free radicals are oxygen molecules that become stressed or split and/or have unpaired electrons. These free radicals cause damage to cells, proteins and DNA and are the beginning of many illnesses and diseases. Lack or diminished production of melatonin can also trigger the aging process. Serotonin is a neurotransmitter, a "happy" chemical, and it is transformed into melatonin in the pineal gland. Some believe that the connection of the pineal gland with its optical cells helps one to "see" and that is why it is called the "gateway to higher consciousness". It is said, when activated, some can "see" through the illusion of this world, which enables them to see into other worlds and dimensions.

Spiritual Significance. The Crown/forehead chakra (third eye vertical) is the center of spiritual consciousness, divine Oneness or Christ, Buddha or Cosmic Consciousness, where one experiences an expanding illumination of divine oneness. In this state, one feels a loving kindness for all, a universal love and a desire to serve ALL. Compassion, direct knowing, direct inner perception, unceasing desire to serve others are traits of one with an awakened forehead chakra. When all the chakras are aligned and working together in harmony AND you are living and being truthful in all aspects of your life (reflected by the pituitary gland), then the probability of awakening your pineal is exponentially increased. When these two glands are electrically charged and connected is when we experience God, Christ, Buddha or Cosmic Consciousness. The pineal gland controls the right side of the brain (intuitive brain), left eye, ear, and left side of the body. This is the chakra of self knowledge.

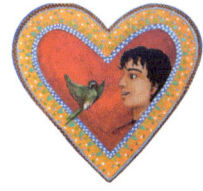

SeeMore and Matisse say, the pineal gland produces only one hormone, melatonin. Melatonin helps run your body's clock for day and night, and the clock for the longer cycle of growth from infant, to child, to adult, to old age. Melatonin also cleans the body of loose damaged cells that if they stayed could develop into illnesses and diseases. The most important thing the pineal gland does is connect us to the higher or expanded realms of being through meditation. Some call it the "God/Creator/First Source" gland because when it is activated through meditation and rightful actions, it can connect you to *God* directly. In higher connected states you just KNOW things (without studying), because you are not separate from anything, you are ONE with everything. Because of this "oneness" feeling, you feel love and have compassion for all life. Direct knowing happens because you realize that you are part of the Divine Infinite and have a soul and that we are Spirit that is only temporarily residing in a body container (in a holographic world).

Part 3 Organs of the Body

Brain: The Nervous System of the Human body
Heart: Circulatory System
Lungs: The Respiratory System
Liver: Digestive System
Spleen: Lymphatic System
Stomach: Digestive System
Small Intestine, Large Intestine (Colon, Rectum, Anus): Digestive System
Gallbladder: Digestive System
Kidneys, Ureters, Bladder and Urethra: Urinary System
Reproductive System:
        Female organs: vagina, clitoris, vulva, uterus, cervix, breasts
        Male organs: penis, testicular sacs, prostate

Please note: Organs, as well as glands are more complicated and intricate within themselves and how they work. They are all interconnected throughout the body. The explanations contained here are basic and further study and investigation is encouraged. Liberty has been taken to present explanations of some of the organs in a non-conventional way. Historically, the magical role that these organs play in our bodies has been either ignored or down-played by many cultures. I have therefore, with respect, made an effort to re-elevate their significance and stature. A less mechanical approach is taken and replaced by an attitude of appreciation and gratitude. Positive attitudes, such as gratitude and appreciation, are important factors in healing. These positive attitudes not only heal the body but also heal the mind and emotions; which allows for the soul's expression to emerge and re-unite with Spirit.

GLOSSARY

Organ is a part of an organism that is self-contained and has a specific vital function, such as the liver and the heart in humans. Organs have specialized tasks and their respective functions are grouped into systems. Examples are: the circulatory system´s task is to circulate blood, which the heart (organ) is instrumental in doing. The digestive system´s task is to break down food into parts that the body can utilize. Some of the organs that accomplish this task are: the stomach, the small and the large intestines. The nervous system´s task is to act as a communication network that connects all parts of the body; the brain, spinal cord and nerves are organs that help accomplish this task.

Chakra means wheel or disk, as in spinal cord discs, where energy or vital life force flows and circulates throughout the body. There are seven main disc energy centers that start at the base of the spine (matter) and circulate up to the crown of the head where the energy meets with cosmic or divine energy consciousness. In the fullest meaning of this Sanskrit word, chakra is when the energy from the lower disc chakras located in the lower spine can travel by meditation and overcoming lower emotions) up to the crown chakra. The whole point is that each of us is divine already; we just need to re-connect matter/body with the higher crown chakra/Spirit. **Yoga** means union of one´s physical, mental and emotional bodies with the soul and universal Spirit.

Torus, is a "donut shaped" field of energy that feeds or generates its own energetic self by rotating its field in a circular movement. The energy starts from the bottom inner ring of the donut, goes through the center (of the donut) and flows upward and outward towards the outside or perimeter of the donut and back and up to and through the center, infinitely repeating these revolutions until the energy dies or transforms into another form. Some torus have smaller thinner centers and some larger; they come in infinite sizes to accommodate the structure of matter. Examples of various sized torus fields around life´s structures are: human body (matter/form), human unique heart (matter/form), every planet (matter/form), all stars (matter/form), every sun (matter/form) and galaxy (matter/form).

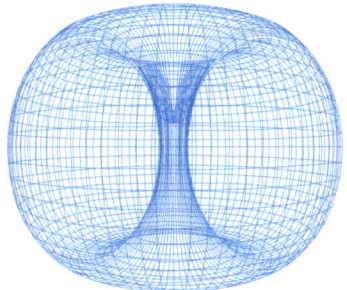

Figure 1. A torus has a "donut" energy field.

The torus fields of the human form (figure 2). The human form has two elecromagnetic torus fields. The one around the body travels through the spinal cord out through the top of the head and continously recirculates. The heart has its own torus field. Both fields gain in strength as we emotionally and mentally mature.

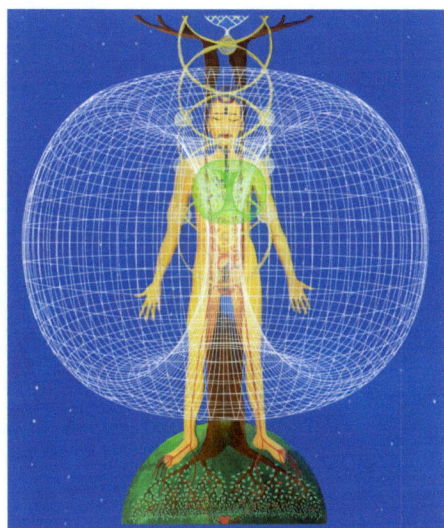

Note: For more information there are YouTube videos available on Flower or Life (in 3D spheres, its flat circular form), and torus fields. Search and find your favorite! Also look up Buckminster Fuller, Nassim Haramein and Dan Winter for more information to explain these geometric structures that energy has as its pattern or blueprint for matter.

Brain: Part of the Nervous System

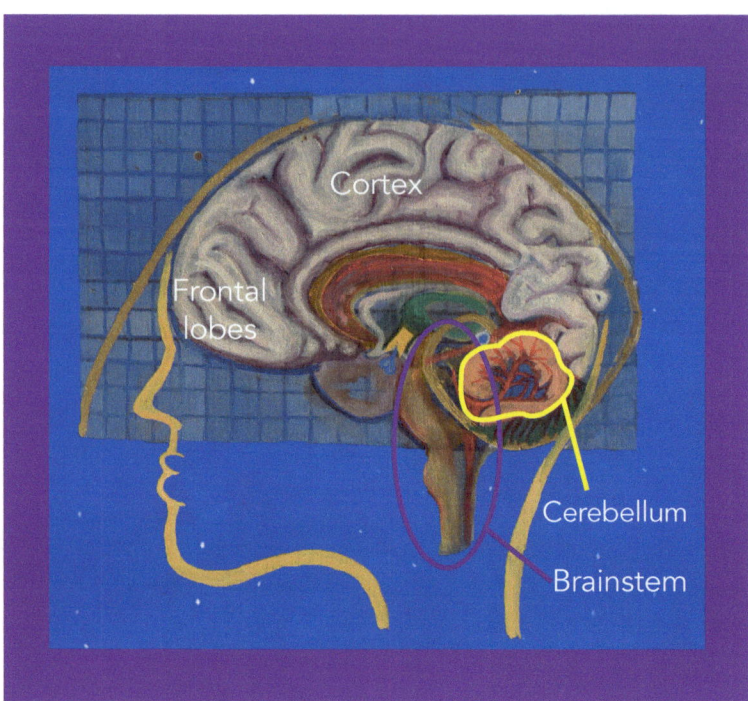

Figure 1. The structure of the head, where the brain is located, is based on the PHI proportion, reflected by the Fibonacci sequence and the Fibonacci Spiral or the Golden Means Spiral.

Location. The brain is located in the head. It consists of a soft convoluted mass of gray and white matter that controls and coordinates the mental and physical actions through electrical current. These currents travel through and are connected to the rest of the body by the spinal cord; from the spinal cord to the nerves that branch out throughout the body in a fractal manner.

Sections of the brain.

The cerebrum includes (1) the upper top section of the brain called the cortex and (2) the forehead or frontal lobe section. These regions, when activated are where higher thinking (problem solving), numerous possibilities and mature or evolved emotions reside. This section of the brain becomes exponentially more active and accessible when integrated with the heart and intuition.

The lower or brainstem portion of the brain is referred to as the first/primitive/or reptilian brain. The brainstem/primitive mind has its corresponding lower to mid range emotional responses, which involve non-thinking, reactive and instinctive responses (lower emotions). The higher or mature or evolved emotional responses are located in the cortex and frontal lobe areas of the brain. The brainstem area includes the following regions: thalamus, mid brain, pons and the medulla.

This section will be devoted to the various conceptions and misconceptions about the brain and are discussed below for your consideration.

The brain is the most complicated and complex of all organs. Our brains are constantly giving us awareness of our environment and ourselves. It does this by continuously processing and providing a constant stream of sensory data. The brain is basically a *perceiver* and *receiver* of information. The information that is received and perceived by the brain is usually influenced by beliefs: personal, religious, political and/or cultural. Information based on beliefs runs a higher possibility of being distorted, swayed or rationalized; usually leaning towards the respective belief. One common way a conflict or *cognitive dissonance* can arise is when the incoming information and the beliefs are not the same. THE primary cause of dis-ease (disease) is the conflict. The body knows when the information received is not "right" or contrary to the belief. To remedy the conflict the ego mind refuses to listen to the perceived information and finds a way to rationalize the information. The body's wisdom is hence ignored. This is the exact point where conflict arises and lives… and many times nurtured by rationalized beliefs.

Another misconception about the brain involves *conception*. The brain does not problem solve nor does it conceive or create ideas. Higher mind resolves and conceives through imagination. Imagination is where creativity resides, not in the intellect. Great minds such as Tesla, Gandhi and Einstein can testify to this, as their ideas did not come from tedious work of the intellect but from inspiration and imagination. The work came after to prove and support the new idea. When one uses the higher mind to conceive, the probability of having non-conflictive perceived and received gathered information is higher. This is the efficiency that can become a part of the process from having a non-conflictive intellect. The freer one is from states of conflict, between beliefs and non conflictive information gathered; the more efficient and useful the intellect can BE in *support* of the new idea conceived in one's imagination.

Therefore, it is of utmost importance that we re-define and re-assign the different jobs of the brain. The brain, based on the dictionary's definition, is the major organ that collects data. So it is a perceiver and receiver of information. Higher mind is conceiver of ideas and it can create through imagination. Re-assigning jobs with this new division of labor, brings clarity and greatly diminishes conflict and unnecessary mental chatter and labor. Conflict and assigning the brain to do the higher mind's job stresses the brain (and body) giving it a job that it is not designed to do. This is the cause of much misery.

After re-defining the brain's tasks, one can become even more efficient by calming the emotions and mind through meditation. All great minds, including the ones mentioned, can testify to this and have included some form of practice of meditation in their private lives. The calmness that evolves through meditation can help one develop more of an observer perspective. The *observer* becomes more aware and objective, as opposed to being subjective and reactive. In the subjective state, minimal and narrow perspective options are available. In the observer state, one becomes more aware of numerous options and wider inclusive perspectives.

Spiritual Significance. The Crown Chakra also includes the upper spine and the entire the nervous system. The brain is controlled by the crown chakra. In the brain are the two most important glands, the pituitary and pineal. When they become charged; higher "Christ" consciousness is achieved. Christ, Buddha, self-realization, illumination and cosmic consciousness all symbolize the same concept. Achievement of this higher state of union (yoga) becomes more accessible when there is a coherency between the intuition and the body (with all its functioning parts: organs, glands and chakras etc.). There must also be a coherency and integration in one's life between the intuition and the emotions and one's actions. These alliances naturally lead to higher consciousness and inclusion. A charge is guaranteed when the following happens: the body, the mind, the emotions and one's soul; along with rightful actions are all coherent and functioning as a unit (yoga). This union within Self can then express the ultimate truth, which is LOVE. Through the crown chakra, feelings of loving-kindness is unconditional and freely given to All (inclusion). Separation (exclusion) is no longer experienced only Oneness. Oneness is ultimately symbolized by our connection to Spirit or cosmic consciousness.

Very important information regarding the Vagus Nerve (See figure 1 brainstem).
One of the cranial major nerves, sometimes referred to as the pseudogastric nerve, starts from the lower/first/primitive or reptilian brain and travels down the body to the lower digestive system. Specifically it includes areas of the mouth (pharynx larynx and soft palate) interfaces with connections to the heart, lungs, liver, stomach, kidneys, bladder, small and large intestines (the entire digestive tract). There are two vagus nerves (located on each side of the body's spinal cord) that have the same exact functions so they are referred to in the singular. The paired vagus nerve accommodates some of the paired glands that are located on each side of the body. Some believe that the vagus nerve actually creates an obstacle in overcoming lower emotions. It can do this because this nerve has fractal branches or tentacle nerves that go into every major system with their accompanied glands and organs. These tentacle nerves directly links and unites them to the primitive or first brain where survival and instincts reside. It is also the place where fear strongly resides.

Heart, Circulatory System, how blood travels throughout the body and more.

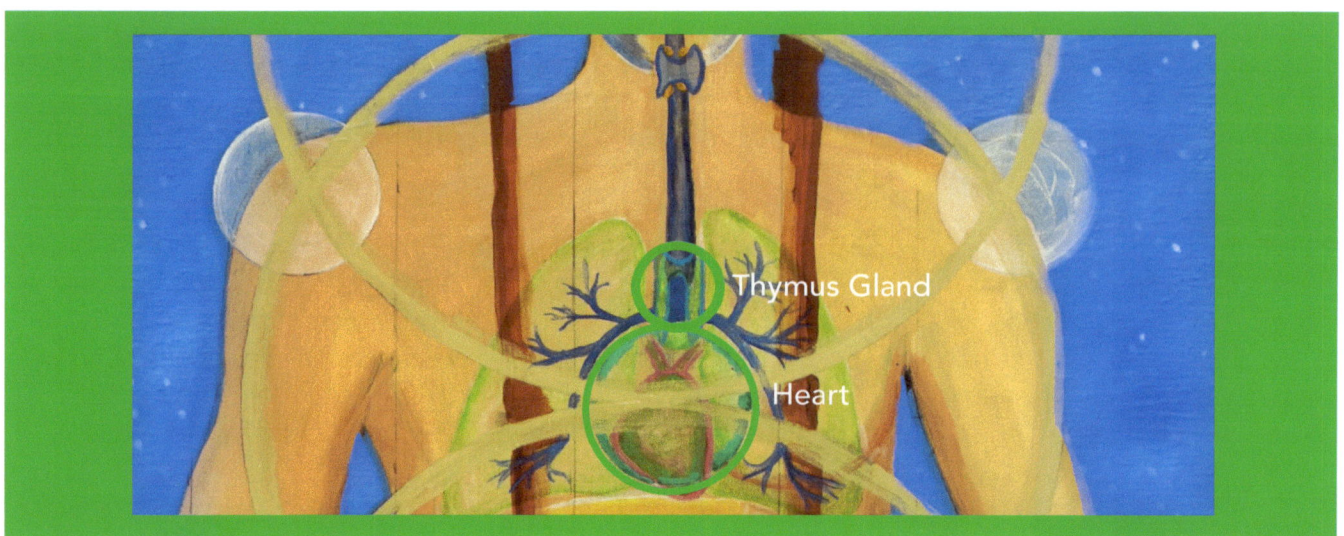

Location. The heart is about the size of your fist and is located slightly to the left center behind chest bone between the lungs. It weighs about 10 to 12 ounces (280-340 grams). It "pumps" about 6 quarts (5.6 liters) of blood throughout the body per minute…that's 2,000 gallons or 7,571 liters a day! There is also a thin membrane *skin* called a diaphragm that separates the upper organs: mainly the heart and lungs from the lower organs: the digestive, urinary, reproductive and lymphatic systems.

Function/how it works. The heart has two sets of four layers of myo-fiber angled muscle tissues each. Each set has two opposing vortices (figure 3): The larger vortex receives blood from the body and sends it to the lungs to get oxygenated. The smaller vortex receives oxygenated blood from the lungs and sends it to the body. The heart does NOT pump blood, like most information claims. It actually sends the blood through an ingenious synchronized valve system that puts a spin on the blood in a vortex spiral action. The actual shape of the valves, its structure and stems, for the arteries and veins all aid in creating a synchronized spin or vortex movement on the blood within the heart. Also when the blood enters the heart, its flow is decelerated by the valves and layered angled muscle tissues as they also aid in putting a spin on the blood. The valves are strategically positioned and spaced and alternately either push and/or suck the blood through the chambers and valve system.

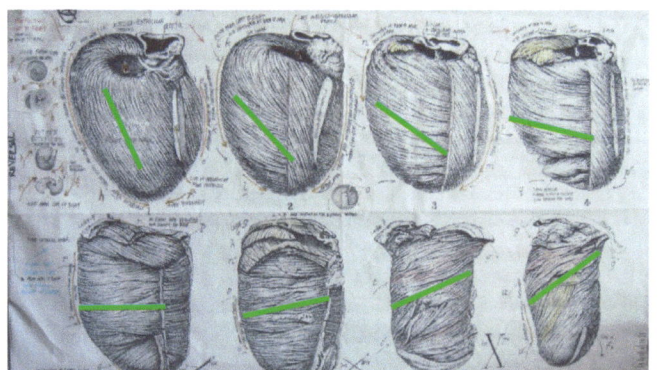

Figure 1. *Title: Fiber angles layers of the Heart and the Etheric 5th chamber by Bradford Riley*

Note: The angles of the muscle tissues are based on root 3, which Frank Chester claims is at 36° (not 45° like others claim). The spiral or spin motion creates the *chestahedron*, which is the result of a balanced integration between the two poles (dualism) of the tetrahedron and the hexahedron geometric forms. See figure 5.

OTHER facts about the Heart
In addition to the valve and angled layered muscle tissues, some sources claim that the invisible lines of the electromagnetic field of the heart further aid in the circulation of the blood, because of its torus-geometric shape. The torus field around the heart is electromagnetic making the heart 100,000 times stronger electrically and 5,000 times stronger magnetically than the brain. The heart is also the FIRST organ to develop in every living thing that has a heart.

Please note: The heart is a very complex organ and there exist many conflicting ideas about how the heart actually functions. This is only one explanation; it is the best I could find at the moment. Further research is encouraged; one day we will know how it actually works!

The heart's valve system works in sync, pushing and sucking the blood in unison at the same time! You can hear it. We have improperly named this action "pumping". The pump sound is actually this *in sync* sound of the valves simultaneously moving the blood by suction and pressure caused by the opening and closing of the valves. The blood is moving into the next section of the heart, lung, and/or body aided by the myo-fiber layered heart muscle, the heart's elecrtomagnetic field and vortexes. SeeMore and Matisse say, "Now that is magical!"

To be used in conjunction with figures 2 and 4A / 4C.
Right side of the Heart. There are two tubes coming to the heart from the body, one from the top called the superior vena cava and one from the bottom called the inferior vena cava. The blood from these two veins is now depleted and needs to be cleaned and oxygenated, so the blood enters the heart. The blood enters the right atrium chamber and fills it. The blood is decelerated by the strong tricuspid valve (4C) as it leaves the right atrium and enters the right ventricle. The blood then leaves the right ventricle through the pulmonary valve (4A), away from the heart through the pulmonary arteries: one goes right and one to the left that leads to each lung. The lungs will then clean and oxygenate the blood.

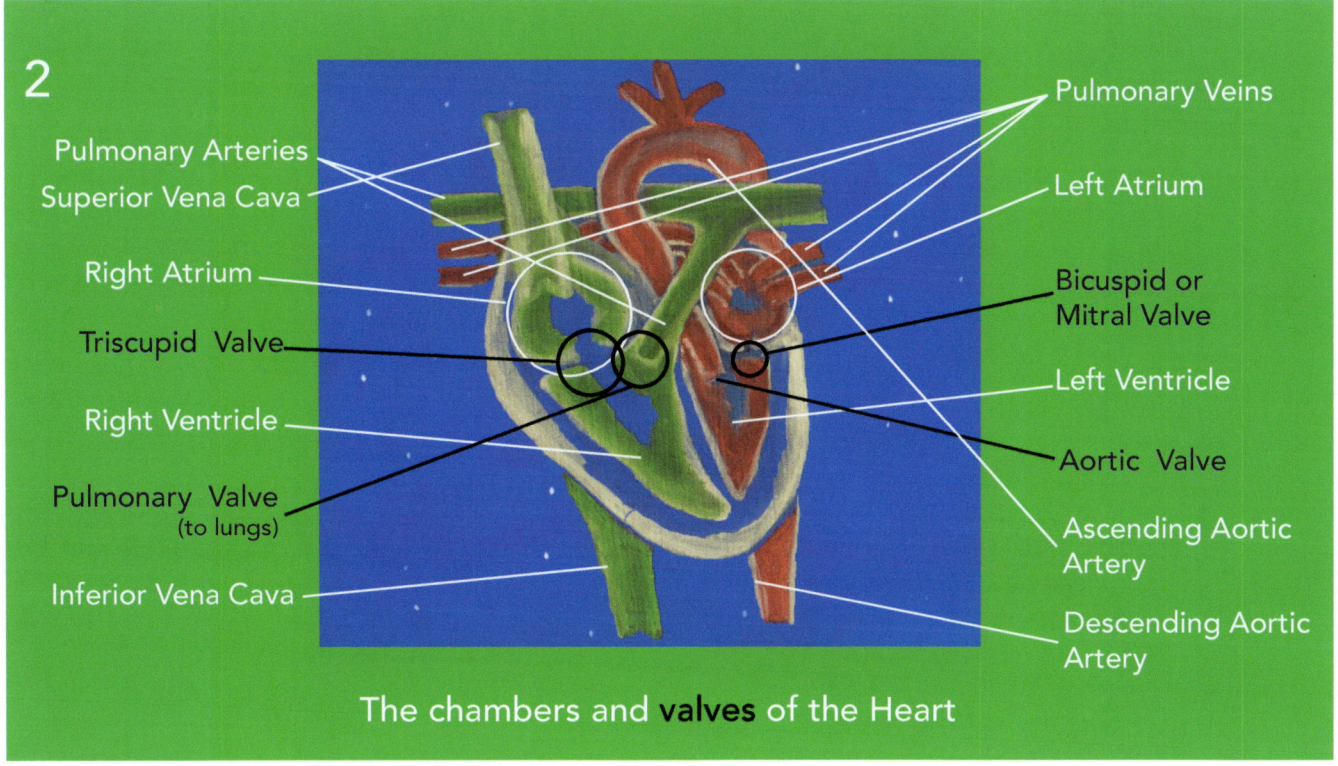

The chambers and **valves** of the Heart

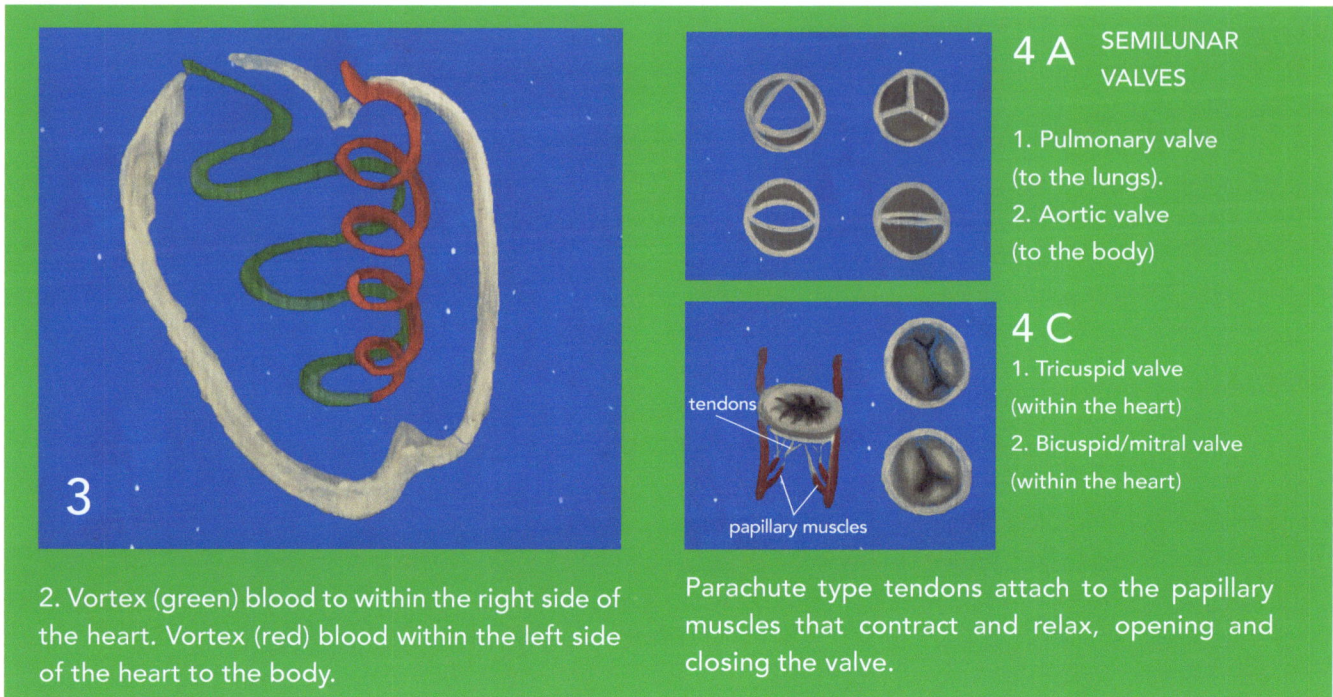

3

2. Vortex (green) blood to within the right side of the heart. Vortex (red) blood within the left side of the heart to the body.

4 A SEMILUNAR VALVES

1. Pulmonary valve (to the lungs).
2. Aortic valve (to the body)

4 C

1. Tricuspid valve (within the heart)
2. Bicuspid/mitral valve (within the heart)

Parachute type tendons attach to the papillary muscles that contract and relax, opening and closing the valve.

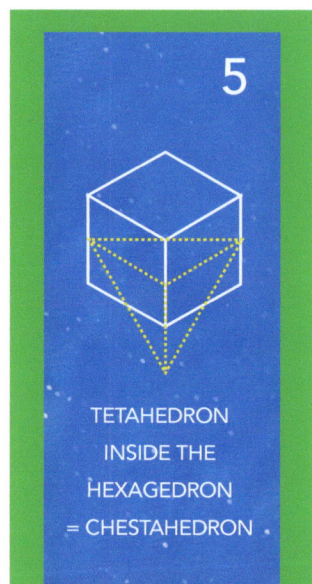

5

TETAHEDRON INSIDE THE HEXAGEDRON = CHESTAHEDRON

Left side of the heart. After the blood receives oxygen from the lungs, the blood re-enters the heart and travels through the pulmonary veins into the left atrium of the heart. From the left atrium the blood leaves through the bicuspid or mitral valves (4C) and goes into the left ventricle. The blood then leaves the left ventricle through aortic valve (4A) and goes into the ascending aorta. The blood then gets distributed to the rest of the body. This cycle repeats itself, *moving the blood in sync* through heart's chambers, valve systems, to and from the lungs, and circulating to all of the body to keep you alive and well without YOU being conscious of it. Again, approximately 2,000 gallons or 7, 571 liters of blood passes through the heart a day; from the body into the heart to the lungs and from the lungs back into the heart out to all of your body!

Valves, veins and arteries. The tricuspid and the mitral or bicuspid valves control the blood from the atriums to the ventricles; chambers within the heart. And the pulmonary and aortic valves control the blood flow out of the ventricles, away from the heart: either to the lungs (pulmonary) or leaving the heart to the body (aortic artery). Veins are elastic elongated tubes that carry blood towards the heart and arteries are elastic elongated tubes that carry blood away from the heart to all the body.

Something Magical: Cymatics.
Cymatics defined: Sound creates a frequency which creates and affects everything, including all life that has form/matter. Sound can be either heard or it is undetected by the human ear. (Watch fun video on YouTube by Nigel Stanford CYMATIC). More information in Part 4.

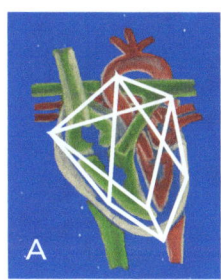 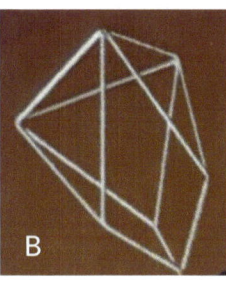 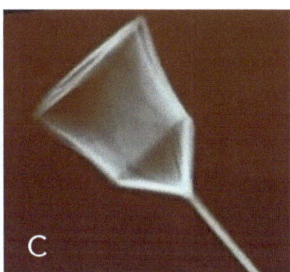

Figure 6 A, B and C. Screenshot YouTube video: Green Meadow Waldrof School. Part 4, Frank Chester heart lecture. October 2009. Time: 2:29 min.

Last words about the "controversial" heart. I think that Frank Chester is on to something, especially when considering that the heart has its own electromagnetic field. I also think that because it has its own electromagnetic field that we can make choices that can affect its frequency, as science is showing through various simple experiments done with sand on a vibrating surface. As the frequency was increased, so was the complexity of the geometric forms. It is therefore not a big leap to conclude that our hearts may be geometric form in motion, which can be influenced by our own frequencies of our personal and collective emotional, mental and spiritual states. In addition to changing the frequencies of our heart vibration he also believes that the heart's structure itself is two basic geometric forms: the cube or hexahedron and the tetrahedron. The tetrahedron is encased within the hexahedron with the tetrahedron slightly protruding from the hexahedron (see figure five). He believes that these two basic geometric forms together create a third form, which he calls *chestahedron* that is positioned at 36 decrees (based on root 3). The heart moves in synchronicity with each beat as the blood goes through each layer of myo fiber tissue. The heart makes a rhythmic pattern or beat; this sound is reflected by the geometry that is in motion: 1) vortexes of the tetrahedron and hexahedron slightly change position as the blood travels through the heart's angled 8 layered myo-fiber muscle tissues (see figure one.). 2) The spin of each vortex as blood enters and exits the heart (see figure three). 3) Synchronized pushing and sucking of the blood as it travels through the valves and chambers of the heart. (see figure two). These actions and their respective motions all-together create another geometric form. He demonstrates this theory by attaching the tetrahedron wired form nestled within the hexahedron wired form and attaches a drill bit to them and proceeds to spin the forms in a transparent bucket of water. As the attached forms spin a 36-decree angle the points of each form creates the third form, the chestahedron. (see figures six A y B). Frank Chester claims that the geometry in motion that becomes visible in the water is a "bell shape". I choose to see it as a chalice! (see figure six C). Could you and I be the Holy Grail (s) we have been searching for?

Spiritual Significance. The heart, lungs, immune system, blood pressure, higher emotions and circulation all belong to the heart chakra both front and back. Their colors are green and emerald green. The physical permanent seed of the soul is located in the heart chakra and in the physical heart. With intention and practice one can feel the presence of this seed, it is a powerful and humbling experience. This chakra is the center of transmutation of the lower self emotions of the solar plexus chakra and higher "universal" oriented emotions of the "higher thymus" heart. Both types of emotions are needed and are equally important in one's spiritual evolution. Self-healing in the lower solar plexus creates space, as well as oportunities where healing can take place with self and others. This action can continue to create even more space, expanding and evolving to include even more people, places, animals, plants and things. As we continue to awaken, more and deeper expressions of the higher emotions will also. Balancing loving kindness with self-interest and the interest of others through the practice of peace, joy, compassion, kindness, consideration, patience and other such higher emotions can attain this. Finding, balancing, developing and incorporating a state of equanimity between: 1) higher and lower emotions 2) between self-interest and the interest of others/universe and 3) between self love and love of others/universal love; are the main objectives of developing the heart chakra.

Lungs: Respiratory System

Location. There are two spongy air filled organs located on each side of the heart within the upper chest cavity.

Function. The lungs take in air through the nose and mouth and travels down the trachea pipe to the lungs. Within the lungs are tree like fractal main branches called the bronchi, that leads to smaller branches called bronchioles, that end in microscopic air raspberry type cluster sacs called alveoli. The alveoli have 2 jobs: the main job is to absorb air and distribute it into the blood. The other job is to destroy airborne irritates: dust, viruses, bacteria and fungi etc. that enter the lungs during breathing. The lungs inhale oxygen and expel carbon dioxide during exhalation. Carbon dioxide is the released waste of metabolism that traveled from the blood to the alveoli. The lungs are covered by a thin double-layered protective skin called the pleura, which also helps keep the lungs lubricated. Studies show that we use only 30% of our lung capacity. Breathing "like a baby," from the belly greatly increases lung capacity. Our health can greatly improve when the lungs can efficiently perform its respective jobs. Studies have shown that the increase in lung capacity can significantly accomplish this. Fully functioning lungs can extend from the collarbone to the diaphragm!

Spiritual Significance. The back of the heart chakra controls the lungs. This area affects the ability to fight disease and it is associated with the immune system. The lungs also work in conjunction with the solar plexus chakra that deals with sensitivity to emotions, stress and tension, which also affects the efficiency in one's immune system. The heart chakra front and back, is the foundation and gateway for activation of the crown chakra. Further discussion of these concepts are in part 4 and 5.

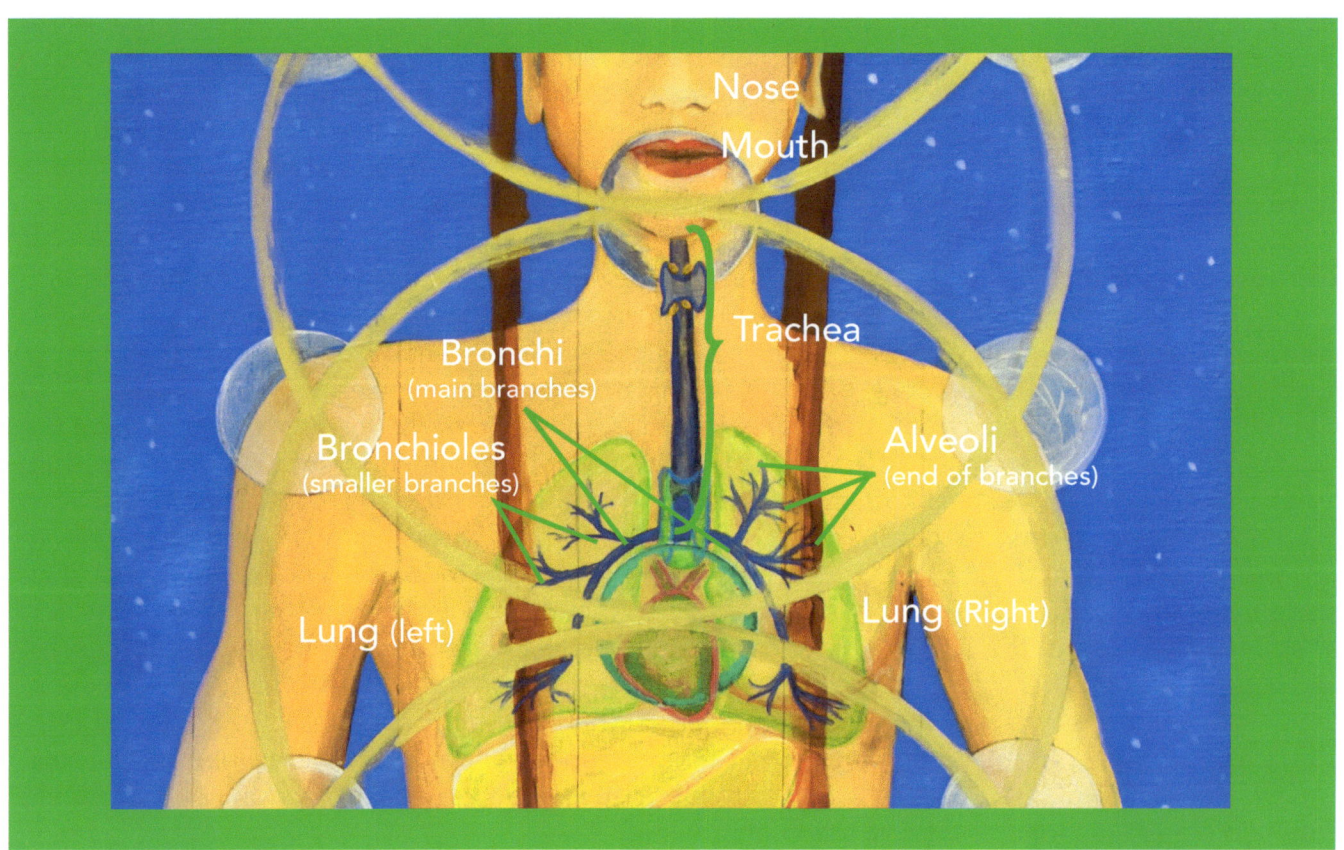

Liver: Part of the Digestive System

Location. The liver is below the heart and right lung and sits on the right side of the stomach. It is protected by the rib cage. It is the body's largest organ and weighs about 3 pounds; it is reddish brown in color. It has four lobes or parts and each receives about 1.5 quarts of blood per minute. It works along with the gallbladder and pancreas, which are right underneath the liver. They all work together with the intestines to digest, absorb and process foods.

Function. Liver's main job is to filter the blood coming from the digestive tract before it goes to the rest of the body. It detoxifies chemicals and metabolizes drugs. The liver secretes bile, which helps break down these mentioned substances. The liver also makes proteins that help clot the blood, converts stored sugar into functional sugar when glucose levels fall, and it destroys old red blood cells.

Spiritual Significance. The liver is associated with the solar plexus chakra. Unregulated lower emotions like anger, stress, resentment, hate and deep-seated hurt all dramatically cause stress on the vital organs of the solar plexus and cause many illnesses and diseases. Therefore proper emotional and mental hygiene is crucial. Hygiene consists of resolving harmful lower emotions. Practicing and developing calm and compassionate emotions with self and others helps to dissipate and alleviate lower emotions. More information is in part 5.

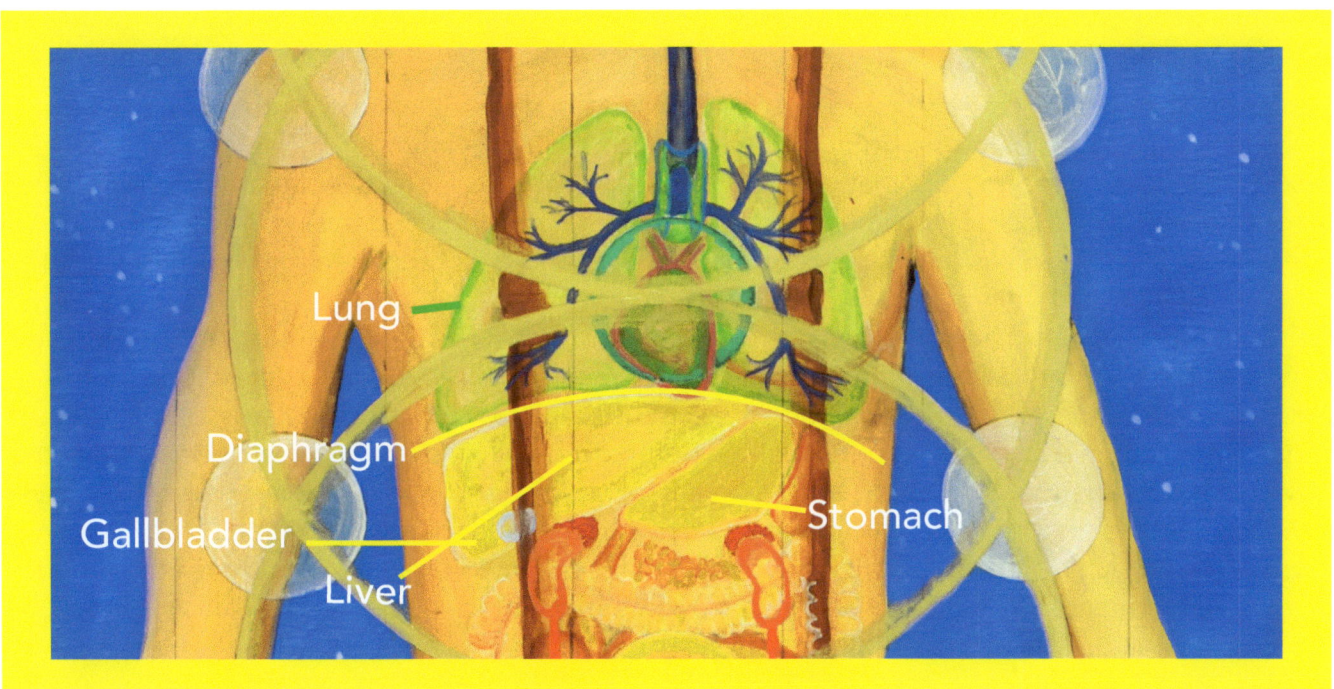

Liver is the large organ on far right. Recall that the diaphragm is the thin membrane that separates the upper cavity that contains the heart and lungs from the lower organs, which start with the liver, stomach and spleen. The diaphragm is flexible and expands as you breathe.

Spleen: Part of the Lymphatic System,
(helps protect the body from foreign germs etc.).

Location. The spleen is located next to the stomach under the rib cage on the left side of the body. Its weighs about 6 ounces, is deep purple in color and it is about 5 inches wide.

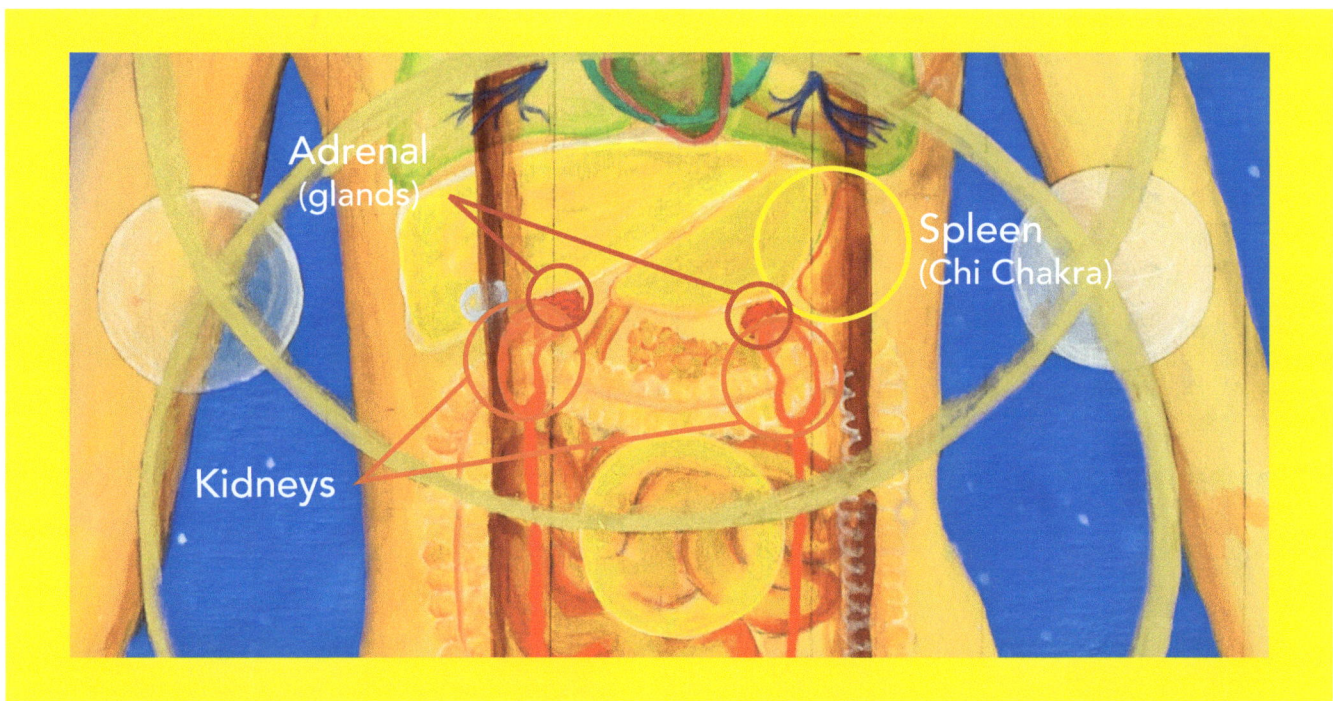

Function. The spleen acts as a blood filter by detecting dangerous bacteria, viruses and other microorganisms that can harm the body. It does this along with other lymph nodes by creating white blood cells called lymphocytes that protect and defend the body. The spleen also controls the amount of red blood cells by letting healthy ones pass through and breaking down old or damaged ones. The spleen has the capacity to expand, creating a storage area for blood.

Spiritual Significance. The spleen has its own chakra located left center bottom of the rib cage front and back. Ancients believed it is the entry point of PRANA, the life energy force, into the body. The condition of the spleen affects the physical and psychological energy of a person. It plays a vital role in a person's general well being and over all strength. As the spleen cleans the blood of foreign germs and viruses, and as one resolves lower emotions and improves their physical and mental diets; the more efficient the spleen can become. Not only will the spleen become more efficient, but it will also enhance the quality of blood. It will enable and increase the amount of vital life force entering the body and insure a more efficient immune system. A highly functioning spleen chakra, also insures an over all stronger naval/CHI chakra.

Gallbladder: Digestive System

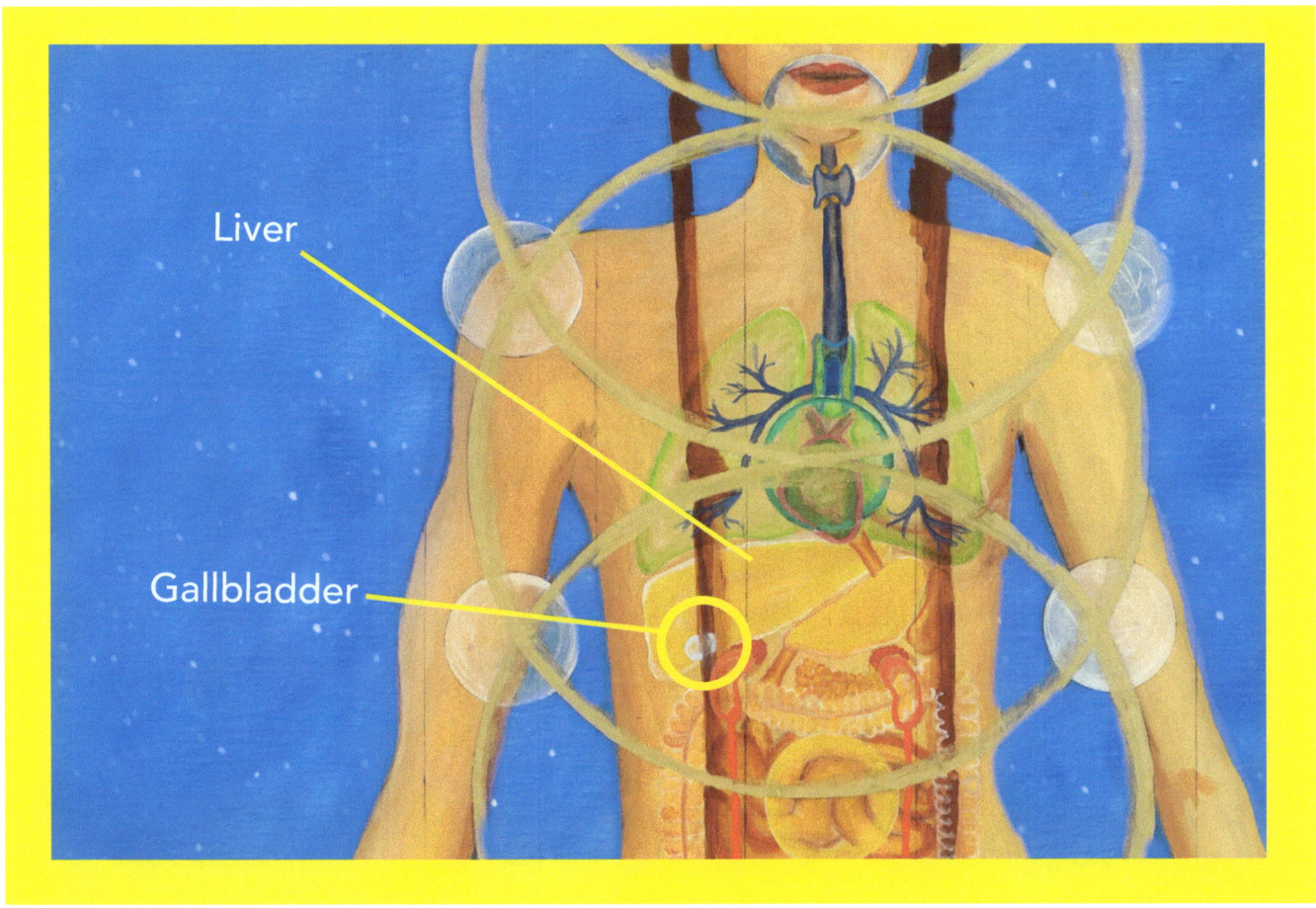

Location. The gallbladder lies posterior under the liver on the right and interior on top of the stomach on the left. It is a hollow pear shaped sac, 3 inches long x 1.5 inches at fullest width.

Function. The gallbladder holds the bile that was made in the liver. Bile is used in the small intestine for breaking down fatty foods. Foods rich in fats and proteins are harder to digest, so bile is needed to help the small intestine. The small intestine can now efficiently extract the nutrients from the fats and proteins that are necessary to feed the cells.

Please note. DIET and your digestive system: For optimum body function, macronutrients are needed by the body and they are proteins, fats and carbohydrates. Fiber rich foods are usually high in carbohydrates. Carbohydrates are the body's main source of energy and they are easiest for the body to digest. Some of these foods are: potatoes (all types) with skin, most beans, most fresh fruits and vegetables, whole grains, nuts and plain yogurts to name a few. Also consider the many studies that validate that when one avoids and/or cuts down on meats, heavily processed grains and added sugars, they can increase their chances of experiencing optimal health.

Stomach: Part of the Digestive System

Location: The stomach is a muscled sac located towards the left side of the abdominal cavity between the liver and the spleen. It is about the size of two fists.

Note: The esophagus is directly behind the trachea, the pipe that carries air to the lungs. The esophagus starts right after the mouth and is the long tube that carries food to the stomach.

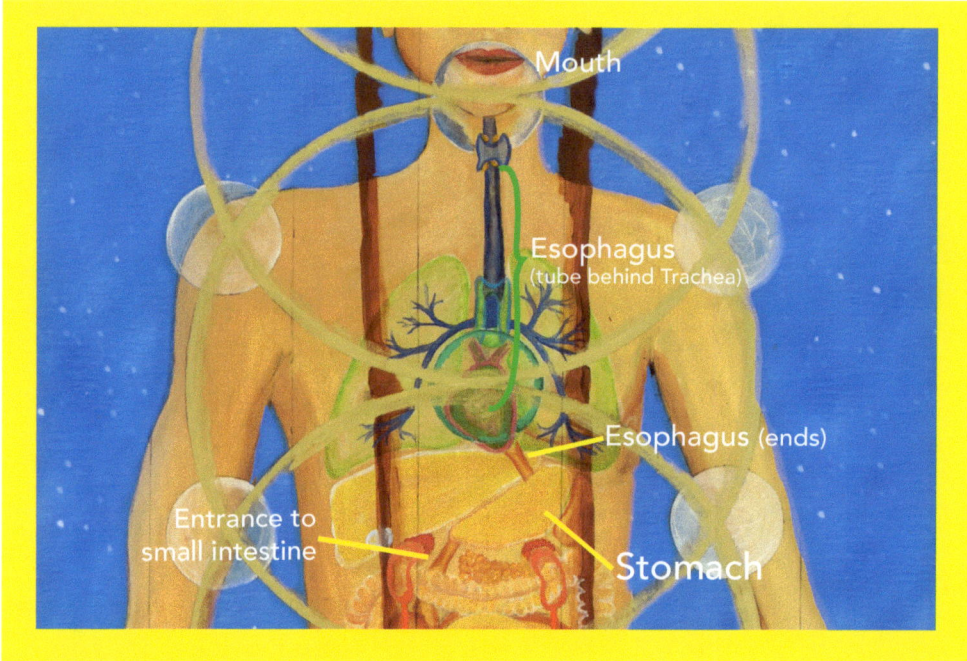

Function. The stomach is part of a group of organs that belong to the digestive system. These organs work together to make food into energy that will feed the entire body. Digestion of food first starts in the mouth when the saliva glands start to secrete saliva to help break down the food. The teeth and tongue also aid in breaking down the food into smaller pieces so it can travel to the throat and down a long pipe called the esophagus that leads and ends at the stomach. The stomach produces special enzymes and acids that further breaks down the food into finer pieces until it has a sludgy consistency. The stomach also acts as a storage tank for food. The sludgy food then leaves the stomach and passes to the rest of the digestive system: the small and large intestines (colon), rectum and the anus.

Spiritual Significance. The stomach is controlled by the solar plexus and navel chakras. These chakras have a two-fold purpose: self will or lower will, which is governed by the masses and the other purpose is higher will, which is governed by the soul. The lower will center shares a dual purpose. One purpose is for developing the positive lower emotions: ambition, courage, perseverance, justice and fairness. The other purpose is to conquer and master the lower emotions: hate, irritation, envy, greed, tension, cruelty etc. Overcoming lower negative emotions and elevating lower positive emotions is paramount in developing coherency between the body, mind, emotions with one´s soul. Incoherency causes havoc on the digestive system in general, especially in the stomach and surrounding organs. When one is in a coherent peaceful state, the organs can more efficiently do their jobs because peace has been established within. Peace within also contributes and establishes a peace that travels out into the environment and world. More information is in parts 4 and 5.

Small Intestine: Digestive System

Location. The small intestine is right below and connected to the stomach. The small intestine is another organ in the digestive system and it involves the *assimilation* of food. It's a long, coiled, small, round tube about the width of one's middle finger and it is about 22 feet (6.7 meters) long!

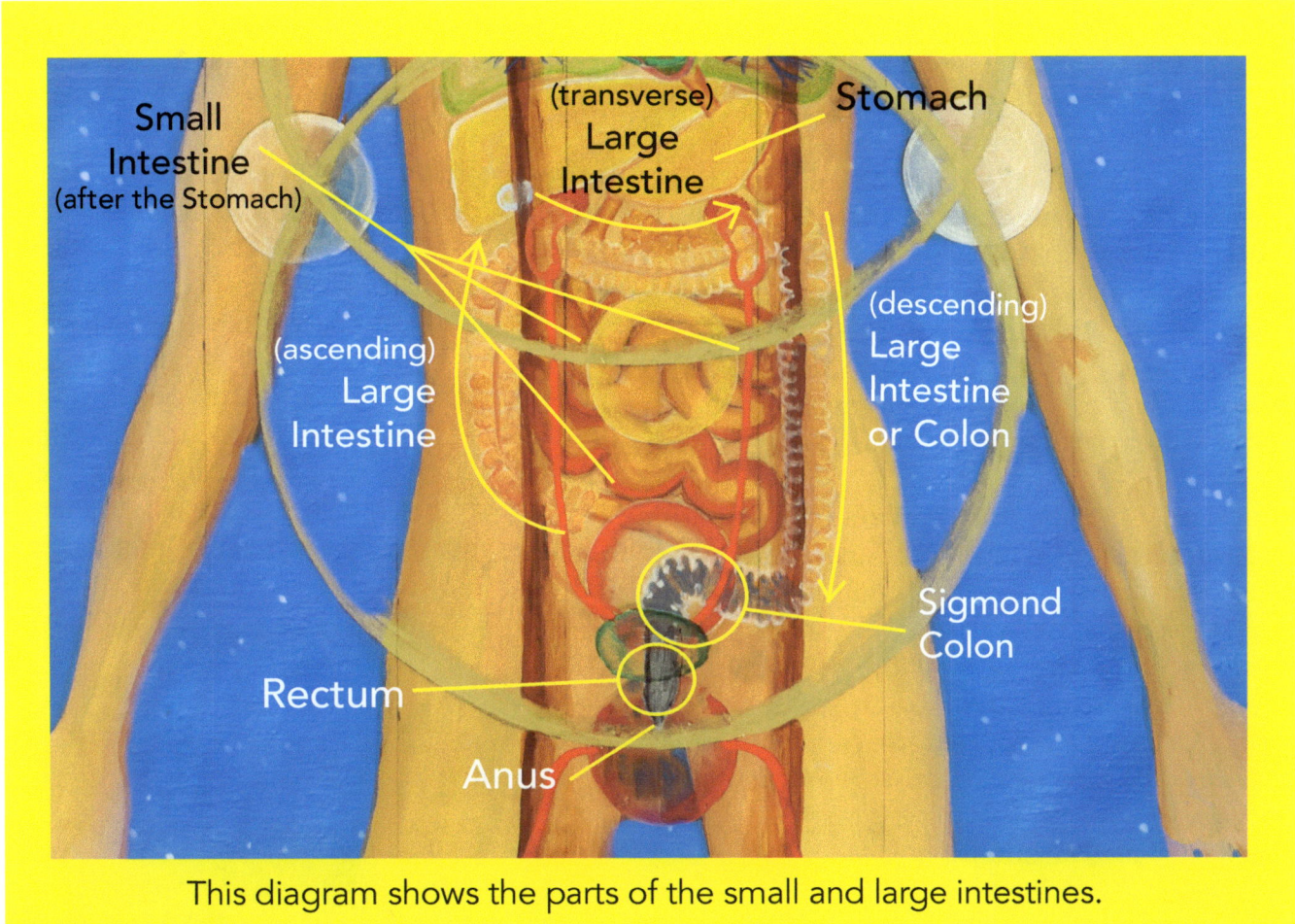

This diagram shows the parts of the small and large intestines.

Function. The small intestine's job to break down food into even smaller pieces, creating a watery sludge that makes it easier for the extraction of fats, proteins and carbohydrates from the food. These extracted nutrients are filtered directly into the blood stream, ready for use as needed or stored in the body. About ninety percent of digestion takes place in the small intestine. The small intestine is divided into three sections. The first section is right after the stomach and is about 10 inches in length. It is called the duodenum. It is within this section that the liver sends in bile and the pancreas sends in pancreatic fluids. These fluids help break down the food, which will be used during the entire digestive process. The second section is called the jejunum. Its is about 3 feet in length and it is where most of the nutrients get absorbed. The third section is the ileum and it is about 6 feet long and it continues to absorb whatever the jejunum did not. The small intestine processes about 2 gallons of food and liquids along with digestive juices that helps to break down the food. The broken down food is called chyme and it is moved through the long intestinal tube by waves of smooth muscle contractions called peristalsis. They begin at the stomach and pass through each section of the small intestine. Each wave is a short distance to allow maximum extraction of nutrients by the villi and microvilli located along the walls of the entire small intestinal wall. The process of moving the chyme from the duodenum to the ileum can take several hours.

Large Intestine also known as the Colon: Digestive System

Please note: that rectum and anus are also included in this section and all share the same spiritual significance along with the small intestine and gallbladder.

Location The large intestine's primary job is the *elimination* of food. It is located and connected directly to and after the small intestine. It is a long smooth tube wrapped around the coiled small intestine. It has three sides: ascending colon (right side of the body), transverse colon (across the body) and descending colon (left side of the body). The large intestine's tube is 2.5 inch (6-7 cm) wide and approximately 5 to 6 feet (1.8 meters) long. It is also another part of the digestive system.

Function. After the usable parts of the food are extracted from the small intestine, the water is reclaimed from the sludge/chyme of the small intestine; salt and any remaining nutrients are extracted by the large intestine. All the rest of the sludge is prepared for exit from the body. After everything can be extracted, the rest is considered useless waste called feces. The large intestine stores wastes in the descending colon.

Descending Colon
The last section of the large intestine.

Location and Function. The descending colon is the largest part of the large intestine and the final part of the digestive system. It is on left side of the body and it includes the last short curve just before the rectum called the sigmoid colon. The muscles along the descending colon walls help squeeze the sludge along. A healthy colon has billions of bacteria that coat the colon and its contents. These bacteria efficiently promote the process of elimination of the sludge or feces to be emptied out of the body.

The rectum is the last stop before the feces is eliminated. The "sludge" is thickened by further water extraction and is mixed with mucous, for easier elimination. It is the actual storehouse of feces waiting for final exit from the body via the anus.

The anus is the very last part of the digestive system or tract. It is a two-inch canal located on the muscles of the pelvic floor. The anus has two sets of round ring shaped muscles called sphincter muscles. One set of muscles is internal, for regulating bowel movements (for sensing when and type of feces). The other set is external, for actual voluntary elimination. The anus sphincter muscles are for the opening (letting out feces) and closing (holding in feces) making elimination possible.

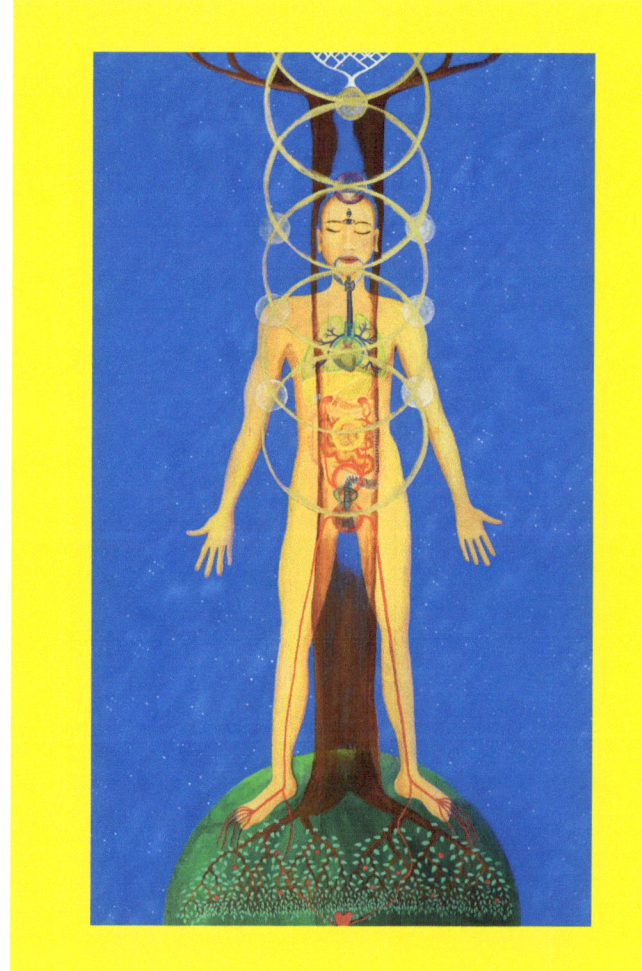

Spiritual Significance of Gallbladder, Small and Large Intestines (Colon) and Rectum

Part 1 Navel and Solar Plexus Chakras and Diets. The small and large intestines, including the colon, rectum and anus, are part of the navel chakra (CHI) system. These organs are also part of the solar plexus chakra, located right above the navel chakra. The CHI or navel chakra also includes additional organs: diaphragm, liver, pancreas, gallbladder and stomach. All of these organs are associated with both chakras because they directly all work in tandem in one of two ways. One-way is aiding in assimilation of foods or converting the food into nutrients, which the body can easily utilize as its source of energy; or the other way involves that the elimination of food wastes. After all the nutrients have been extracted from the food, the remnants or left over part of the food needs to be eliminated from the body. Proper elimination is insurance against contamination within the human body. Nutrients or intake of live food is "prana", which means food is life giving. Intake of healthy life giving foods, directly affect the assimilation and elimination processes of the body. Dead, overcooked, heavily processed foods and excessive meat consumption lack vital force and can cause stress on the organs. Unmanaged stress leads to illness and disease. There is also a mental, emotional and spiritual intake that can feed the whole body or not. Therefore the responsibility not only extends to intake of life giving foods; but to the intake of mental, emotional and spiritual foods that can feed and uplift the human spirit and way of being. One's diet of television, films, literature and use of electronic devices etc. is just as important as the food you put into your body.

Part 2 The affects of the emotions on solar plexus and navel chakras.
The basic emotion of the navel chakra has to do with and centers on CHI. One's CHI is your instinctive power and direct instinctive knowing. It is also the center of strength and assertiveness. When the lower emotions of the solar plexus have evolved, the CHI becomes the golden ball of light energy that has the potential to travel through the spine up to the higher chakras. This action accelerates and empowers one's spiritual evolution and can literally make or actualize "Heaven on Earth". This is the same CHI that the martial arts refer to as the "Golden Ball of Energy". It is the self's source of power. CHI strengthens the body, as it prepares and enables it to manage even more power and higher spiritual experiences. But the CHI/navel chakra works in tandem with the solar plexus chakra, located just above the navel chakra. The solar plexus chakra deals directly with 1) the lower inferior emotions: anger, irritation, hate, envy, greed, violence, aggressiveness, addictions, cruelty, resentment, worry and anxiety etc. and 2) it also deals with the higher (lower) emotions: perseverance, courage, trust, strength and lower/self will. The harmful lower emotions can literally eat away at the digestive and lymphatic organs causing irreparable damage and/or cause interference with their respective tasks. As one evolves and emotionally matures, the lower negative energy dissipates creating a stronger CHI or navel chakra as well as stronger solar plexus chakra. The alliance between these two chakras provide for a strong spiritual base. It can also provide a secure passage for further purification of the lower emotional energies as they travel up the spine to the heart chakra and above. This is where they can finally be released with and in Love. The activation of higher chakras depends on one´s healthy emotional maturity and the purity of vital energies that come from the lower charkas.

Part 3 The affects of using the higher (lower) emotions to overcome lower emotions.
The higher (lower) emotions of this chakra are: ambition, lower will, courage, perseverance, justice, fairness, trust and strength. One has access to these emotions directly in this same chakra and can use them to help over come the lower emotions that also reside in this chakra. Contemplation in using the higher lower emotions to overcome a lower emotion starts when "I" or self begins to separate from the mass consciousness mentality of the solar plexus chakra and desires to evolve

into the higher alignment. The higher alignment is simply reflected in this following statement, "my will be done" evolves into, "THY (God or First Source) will be done". A change of *will*, from self (exclusion of others) for God or Higher Intelligence involves inclusion of others, All. In addition to a change of will is the direct use of a higher lower emotion (such as perseverance) to overcome a lower emotion (such as anger as Matisse does in part 4). As one perseveres and successfully overcomes the anger, they will notice that this chakra will start to connect and align itself to a higher chakra, the heart and above. This is "active intelligence" or intelligence in motion. Intelligence in motion is extremely useful not only in overcoming lower emotions but also the negative effects that the lower emotions had on the body. Higher alignments with the higher chakras calms the organs, glands and body in general, dissipating the constriction and re-active, out of control whims of the lower emotions. As one no longer *feeds* the lower emotions in thought or action, they subside. The freer one becomes from the lower emotions, the more space is created to allow for expansion into the higher chakras, simultaneously disempowering the lower emotions. This is active intelligence in motion as it further reinforces and awakens the *active intelligence* that already existed and exists within each of us now.

Kidneys: Part of the Urinary System

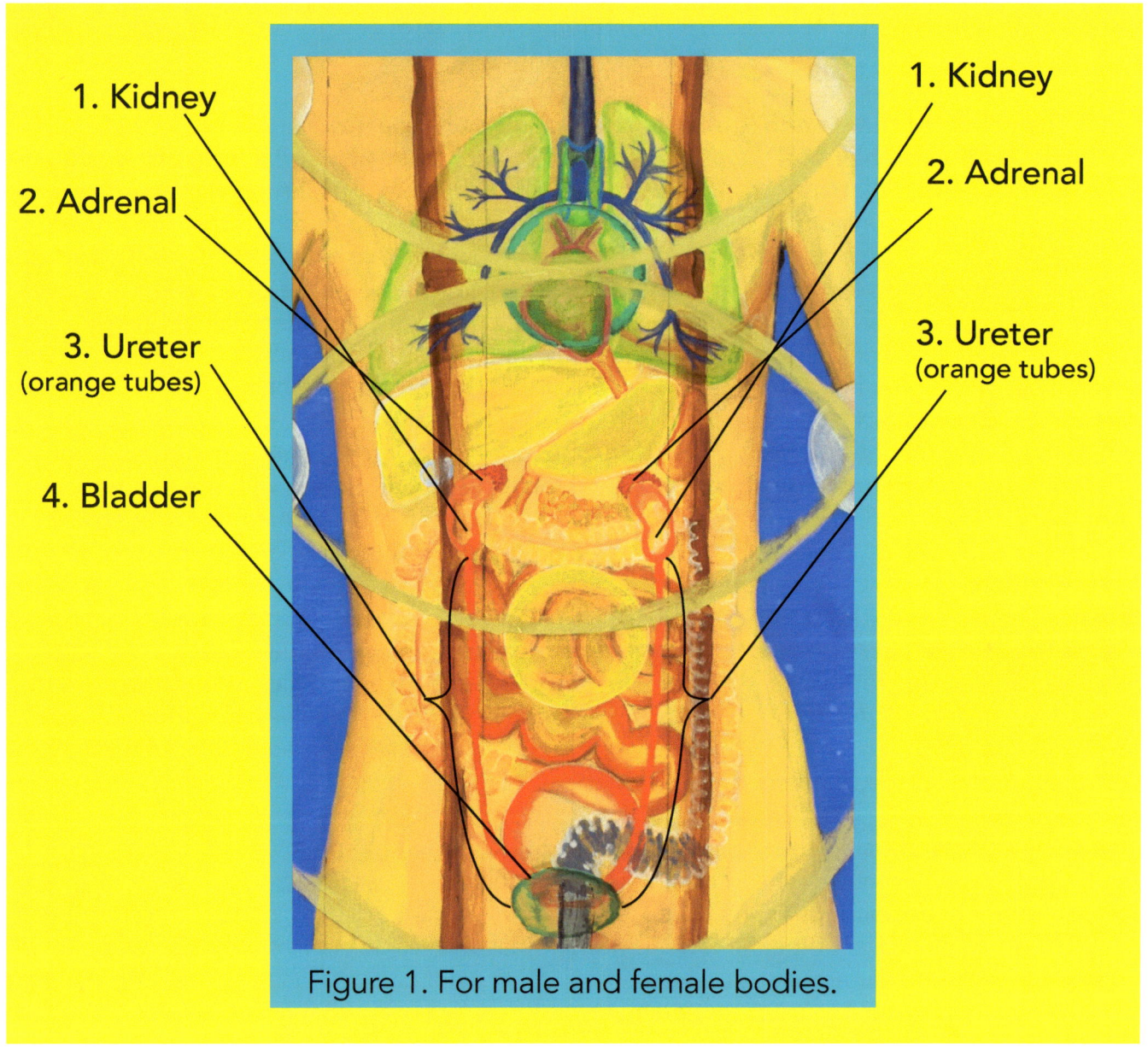

Figure 1. For male and female bodies.

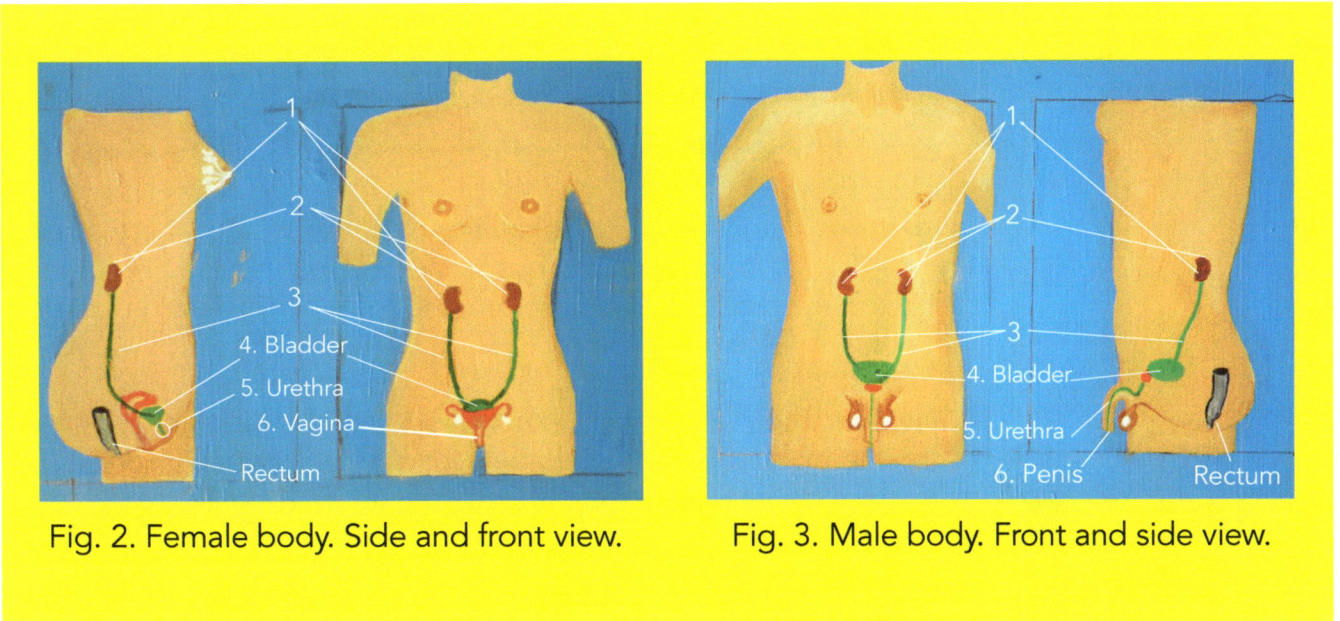

Fig. 2. Female body. Side and front view. Fig. 3. Male body. Front and side view.

Location. There are two kidneys each located on the right and left sides of the spine against the back muscles in the upper abdominal area, protected by the last or 12th shortest rib. They are bean shaped and the approximate size is 11 cm x 7 cm x 3 cm. The adrenal glands sit on top of each kidney.

Function. See figure 1. The kidneys work with two other organs, ureter and the bladder. The kidneys are connected to the bladder by long funnel shaped tubes called ureters. The kidney´s job is to clean the blood by filtering out toxins and other wastes: food, medications and toxic substances. The wastes in the kidneys is called urine. The urine travels to the bladder via the ureter tubes.

More specifically, the kidneys filter the blood before it goes back to the heart. They maintain overall fluid balance within the body and it also regulates and filters minerals from the blood. The kidneys can also function as a gland, creating hormones that help produce red blood cells, promote bone health, and regulates blood pressure and electrolytes. Drinking plenty of clean pure water greatly enhances well functioning kidneys.

Bladder or Urinary Bladder and the Urethra:
Part of the Urinary System (See figures 1, 2 and 3 for kidneys)

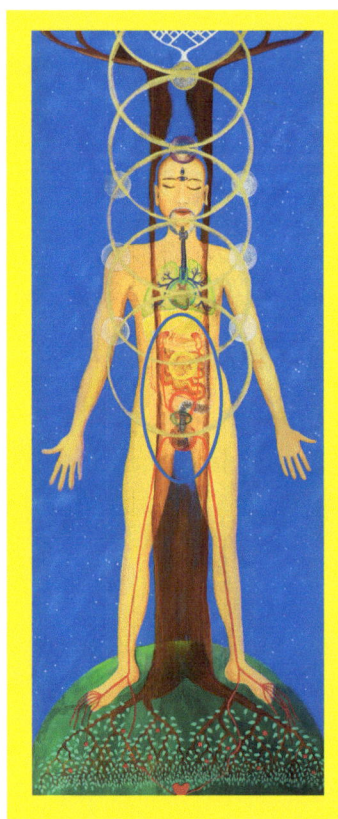

Location. The bladder is located in the lower abdominal area near the pelvic bones.
In females it is in front and below the uterus or womb where a baby grows (fig. 2). In males it sits just above and behind the pelvic bone (fig. 3). The bladder is also in front of the rectum, which is the last portion of the descending colon.

Function. The bladder is an expandable muscular sac, like the stomach. The bladder is connected by a long tube from each kidney. The tubes are called ureters that are approximately 10 to 12 inches or 25 to 30 cm long in an adult. The ureter tubes carry urine that was made in the kidneys to the bladder sac. When the bladder becomes full of urine, it leaves the body through the urethra. The urethra tube that comes from the bladder in women is short and its opening is between the vagina and clitoris, located between the lips of the inner vulva (fig. 2). For males, the urethra tube is about 8 inches long beginning at the bottom of the bladder and ending at the tip of the penis (fig. 3). For urination to occur (for males and females), the bladder muscles contract, signaling the two sphincter muscles to open and let the urine out. When urination is finished the sphincter valve muscles close until the next time urination occurs.

Spiritual Significance. The kidneys, the adrenal glands and the rest of urinary system: bladder, ureters, urethra and blood pressure are all under the control of the Meng Mein chakra. The Meng Mein chakra is approximately 1/2 to 1/3 smaller than the main chakras. Its colors are tones of orange and a little red. The purpose of this chakra is to act as a pump in distributing *prana*, or life energy, to all parts of the body. When we transmute lower dense energies into spiritual energies, *prana* is allowed to flow more easily. The Meng Mein chakra also works in conjunction with the sex chakra and the spleen chakra. Transmutation is the process or journey of evolving the self by using the following tools: self discipline, contemplation, self-analysis and meditation. These tools do two things: 1. help overcome lower emotional energies and 2. help develop higher emotions. Each of these two components enhances and reinforces the other. This is true healing. The healing of the lower emotions transmutes or changes lower emotional vibrational energies into the higher emotional vibrational energies…eventually we learn to BE in the heart chakra and above, while supported and nounished by the energies from the lower chakras. As this process evolves, the prana or life energy becomes more fluid. This fluidness of *prana* actually heals, energizes and vibrates harmony within one's own body. From the body it emanates out and can help heal the environment. The journey of transmutation of the emotions is a moment-to-moment, day-by-day commitment towards making better choices that are more in harmony within one's self, more harmonious towards the environment and all others that live in that environment. This harmonious energy will eventually include the entire planet and the universe… simply because we're all connected.

Male and Female Sex Organs
The physical center for procreation is located in the sacral chakra.

Please note: Some of the female and male parts are organs and some are glands. To more fully comprehend the functions, the glands and the organs (both male and female) are discussed independently and interdependently. I have also included the physical union of male and female bodies for the purpose of procreation. Discussion of sexual union is for procreation purposes only.

As you may recall, the gonads are glands because they produce hormones that carry specific genetic instructions or codes. The male body's gonads are the testes. The testes are where the sperms are made (fig. 2). Each sperm has ½ of the genetic code that is made up of male and his ancestors. The female body's gonads are the ovaries (fig. 1). The ovary is where the eggs are stored. Each egg has ½ of the genetic code of the female and her ancestors.

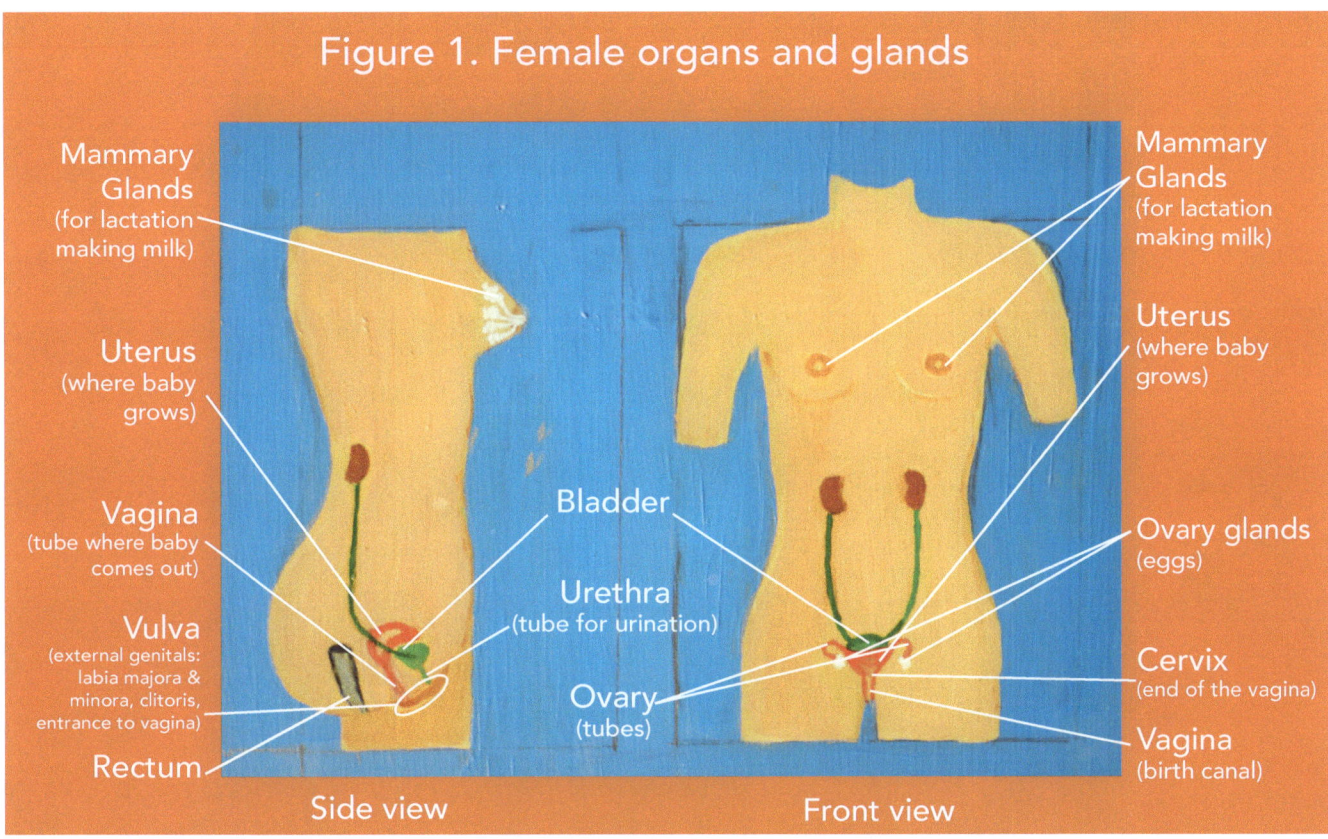

Female Body: Organs and glands described independently.

In a female body, there are two curved ovary tubes that extend from each top side of the "V" shaped pubic area. It is best to describe the female organs from puberty on, as their functions will make the organs and their roles more understandable, creating a clearer picture of procreation and what it means. In puberty, between 10 -13 years old, the female will begin her menstruation. Menstruation is when an unfertilized egg travels through the ovarian tube from the ovary and falls into the uterus; the uterus will recognize that the egg is not fertilized. The unfertilized egg will cause the lining that is in the uterus to break away from the uterine walls causing a female to menstruate, the monthly bleeding that flows out through the vagina. Menstruation only happens during the reproductive years, which begin with puberty and end with menopause, which is usually between 45 and 55 years of age.

The body will discard the lining along with the unfertilized egg. They will travel out through the cervix, down the vaginal canal, to out side of the body approximately every 28 days or so. Each ovary will take turns and release an egg, every other month. Every month the uterus will create and then discard a new rich blood lining made for a potential new life, until an egg becomes fertilized in the uterus, which is pregnancy. When a woman does become pregnant, it means an egg became fertilized and the uterus recognizes this. All the lining that was in the uterus stays and nourishes the growing baby. The woman will not menstruate until sometime after the baby is born, which is usually nine months, or longer (sometimes) if she breast feeds her baby.

Male Body: Organs and glands described independently.

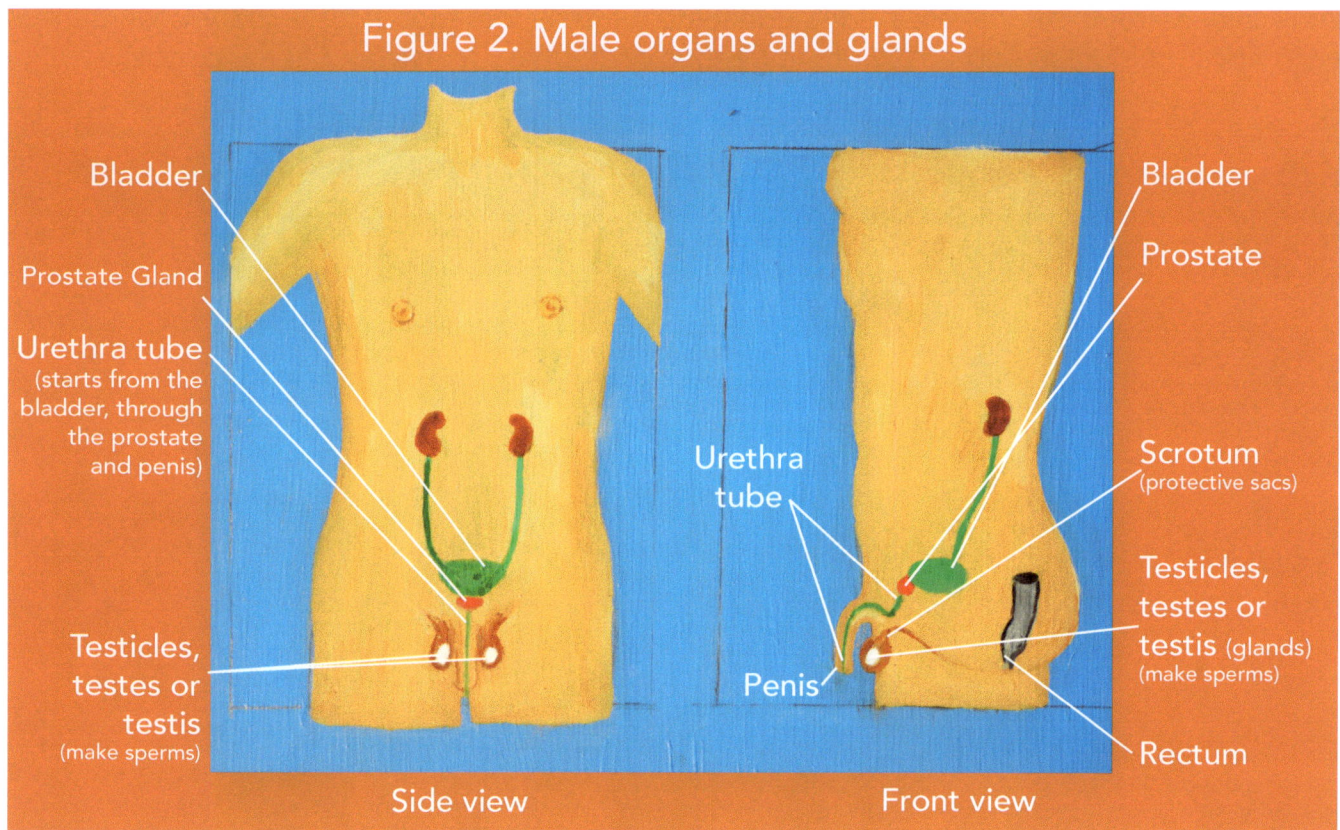

In the male body the male organs are mostly external, outside of the body. The penis is a male organ that has three parts: the part that attaches to the wall of the abdomen is the root. The shaft is the second part and it is the tube where urine and semen travel through. The tip or head of the penis's tube is where the tube ends at the penal opening; it is where the urine and the semen are expelled. The penis is covered by loose skin called foreskin, unless it is removed in a procedure called circumcision. Inside the cylinder shaped tube of the penis are three circular shaped chambers that are made up of sponge like tissues that can be filled with blood to make the penis rigid. On each side of the penis there are two sacs, which is the third part of the male organs, and they are called   the scrotum. They are the loose, pouch like sacs of skin that surround each testicle. The scrotum act as a cooling system to protect the testicles within them. The testicles, testis or testes are large olive shaped glands. The testes produce the sperm and the semen. Semen is the fluid that carries the sperm. The testes also make the hormone testosterone that will become activated in puberty, between 11-14 years of age.

Testosterone is a male's primary sex hormone that generates or produces sperm. The prostate is a gland located right under the bladder and it produces the fluid that nourishes and transports the sperm. The prostate gland has two tubes that connect to each testes. The tube starts in the testes and travels up and around the bladder and enters the topsides of the prostate. The prostate is where the semen is released as it mixes with the sperm as they both travel through the urethra simultaneously.

Procreation: organs and glands of female and male are described interdependently.

Procreation is described in three stages: Stage1, prelude to procreation. Stage 2, sperm and the egg meet. Stage 3, after the sperm and egg meet. Suggested reading: around puberty or when asked.

Stage 1 Prelude to procreation.
Puberty and what it means. It is known that without the charge of desire or arousal, procreation or making babies would not occur. Nature has therefore provided a way to make sure that continuation of the species is guaranteed. This guarantee are the hormones. The primary hormones that first give their *signals* are the pituitary and pineal glands located in the brain. These glands say when it´s time to start puberty and accordingly activate the secondary hormones, which are located in the gonads: testes in the male and ovaries in the female. ALL the hormones begin their respective degrees of secretions at this time and officially start puberty. Puberty is a process where a child's body matures into an adult body. This process is the preparation and maturation of the human body that eventually enables it capable of procreation or of sexual reproduction. Puberty can begin between the ages of 9-13 years. Each individual is unique as to when it comences and it can continue until the ages of 17-21. There are many signs that puberty has begun and that different hormones are at work or activated: females will grow breast and start their menstruation. Males grow bodily hair, their voice deepens and muscle mass develops. The activation of puberty also stimulates and activates many different emotional feelings, including those of wanting to experience independence, degrees of separation from parents, curiosity about the world and curiosity about the opposite sex etc. and there are many more.

The combination of emotional and bodily changes that take place creates a desire. This desire eventually evolves in time where the male will "want" to have union with a female and the female will want to have union with the male. The "want to" is the "guarantee" that nature has provided to insure the continuation of the species. The "want to" is the desire that develops and happens because the sexual organs, with all their nerve endings, have become activated and sensitive by the release of the hormones. These major body organs, as well as other parts of the body, become more sensitive to touch and are capable of becoming aroused. The combination of being physically aroused plus the corresponding emotional response (which is to unite), can evolve into an increase in desire for union. The basic sensitive area for the male is the penis, and the similar sensitive area is the vulva, specifically the organ called a clitoris, for females. The clitoris is a small elongated part of the female genitals at the upper end of the vulva. Arousal stimulates and motivates one into the act of making love or having sexual intercourse, that makes babies. This type of arousal that was just explained, mainly involves the basic corresponding and interdependent organs of the female (the vagina and clitoris) and the male (the penis/prostate).

BUT arousal is much more complicated and can occur in many different ways, which includes kissing, hand holding, intimate conversation, carressing and sensual touching to name a few.

Stage 2: The meeting of sperm and egg.
Author's Note: Below, only the physical aspect of sexual union is explained. But it should be understood and considered that there are many emotions associated with the act of making love or having sexual intercourse. The way we refer to this act shows or reflects our emotional response and maturity about sexual relationships. Basically, it is important to treat others as you would like to be treated. Being responsible to your own body in all its wonders, expressions and capacities and being able to transmit that respect to one's partner is a harmonious way of being.

Commonly, when arousal occurs desire follows and the chance of physical union rises. This "union" has many names: making love, sex, coitus, sexual intercourse etc. and they are all names representing the same act that involves rhythmic movements that unite the penis from the male's body with the vagina from the female's body. Explained in more detail, the vagina has an opening on the outside part of the body, this is one end of the vaginal canal and it is where the penis enters. When a couple is stimulated or aroused sufficiently, the penis (organ) will become erect and rigid. The penis is rigid as you recall, because the 3 spongy chambers in the penis are now absorbed with blood, making it possible for the penis to penetrate and enter the vagina of the female. The desire is the initiation of the union of the penis and the vagina and it is the guarantee that enables the sperm and egg to unite during the act of making love (as described above). The sperm (from the testes) and the seminal fluid (from the prostate gland) of the male, mixes in the urethra tube located inside the penis and comes out of the penal opening. Sometime during the couple's union accompanied by rhythmic movements, the man will reach an excited point called a climax, which a woman experiences also, his penis will then ejaculate that sperm into the woman's vagina. The sperm will swim up the vagina passing through the cervix into the uterus looking for the egg. There are thousands of sperm trying to find the egg. Once one sperm enters (with the assistance of 11 to 13 other sperm) and fertilizes the egg, a protective shield will go up around the egg to prevent other sperm from entering and fertilizing it.

Stage 3: After the sperm and egg meet.
The union of the egg and sperm in the uterus during fertilization becomes a zygote.
A zygote means ½ of the DNA from the father's sperm and ½ of the DNA from the mother's egg formed a new life. The vagina is a tube: at one end is the entrance that has its opening at the outside of the body, other end of the vagina is inside the body and it ends at the cervix. The cervix is the entrance to the womb or uterus. The uterus is where the zygote evolves into a fetus, which evolves and grows into a baby. The cervix is a very strong ring shaped muscle called a sphincter muscle. This type of muscle is so strong it can hold and keep a growing baby within the mother's uterus without it falling out. A baby takes about nine months to fully develop. Once the baby has fully developed, the cervix loosens and stretches. The loosening and stretching of the cervix is called dilation. At this same time, the pituitary and pineal glands are also activating the milk ducts within the woman's mammary glands to produce milk for her baby. When the cervix is fully dilated, about 10cm, the baby will come out into the world through the vagina (also known as the birth canal). When the baby is born the milk is ready.

Author's note. As stated earlier, this topic is explained solely in the context of procreation, which includes only one aspect of our physical form. But human beings are more complex and have mental, emotional and spiritual aspects of their being. Institutions, religions, cultures and some of our laws try to regulate the sexual aspect of our lives. This book does not address any of those other aspects but realizes and respects another's choice. The purpose here is to give an overview and address the different stages of procreation by *connecting (some of) the dots*. Hopefully this *connecting* will provide some answers for our youth. This is only a starting point.

Spiritual Significance. The sex or sacral chakra is located below the stomach and navel. The sacral/ sex chakra controls the sexual organs, bladder, urethra and it also affects the legs, throat and head. Its colors are tones of orange with some red. It is closely related to the base chakra, which is located in back of the body at the tip of spine. This area is where the *kundalini* energy of one's body is grounded to the Earth and the material world. As we sexually awaken during the process and progress of puberty, this energy rises and activates our capacity to procreate.

This tremendous energy can be the *food* that can be utilized and transmuted as it travels up the spine nourishing the higher creativity zones located in the chakras from the heart and above. It is said that a healthy sex chakra is needed for spiritual development because it takes a tremendous amount of energy to evolve or transmute or change the lower frequencies of the lower chakras into higher frequencies of the higher chakras. To transmute sexual energy does not mean suppress or subdue sexual energy. To change or alter the nature of, or transmute sexual energy is to redirect and utilize this energy for other higher chakra purposes. Developing and maturing one's mental, emotional and spiritual capabilities requires discipline and an abundance of energy. This chakra provides some of this needed energy.

Transmutation can only take place if one has a *healthy* attitude towards one's body and sex, where the energy can move freely, unencumbered and successfully up the spine. Also when the lower energies evolve and expand; love and interest only in *self* and a few, transmutes or transforms into universal love for All. This kundalini and sex chakra lower energy can only be transmuted into higher frequencies when and as it moves up into the higher chakras via the spine. As it travels, this energy can also heal and maximize the functions of the organs and glands of the physical body. It also heals, connects and maximizes etheric fields of mental, emotional and spiritual self. These connections also elevate the *quality* of union, as opposed to quantity of unions, when one engages in *making love* or having sexual union.

The higher chakras is the *meeting place* where the lower purified energies coming from the kundalini base, sex (or sacral), navel (CHI) and solar plexus chakras support, connect and mix with the energies of the higher frequencies of the heart, throat and crown chakras. These energies connecting can become even more powerful when they continue up into the incarnated soul, soul, directly to Source/God. When we are capable of uniting the material body with our ethereal (auric) fields by raising our consciousness AND connect it with the Divine, we have Self realized or awakened. We individually have made our contribution to the collective and have created "Heaven on Earth". When the tremendous combination of the following: kundalini energy, healthy sacral (sex) energy and one´s unique CHI energy are all moving in the same direction, our spiritual development and evolution is greatly maximized.

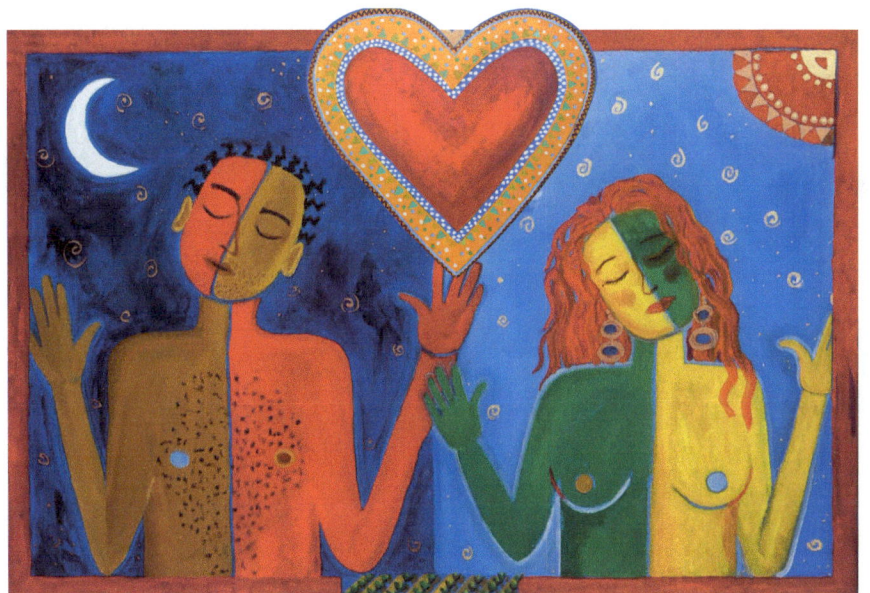

Part 4 Frequency Waves (Hertz) and Light Waves (nanometer) Spectrums

    Full (known) Spectrum
    Our Spectrum
    Frequency, Waves Length and Proton Scales
    In music
    Vibration and the Spectrum in Human Emotions

Part 5 Ancient Schools of Wisdom

    Kabbalah and the 13 Sephiroth
    The Three Pillars of Life
    Inverted Tree of Life

Famous Quotes

If you want to know the secrets of the universe, think in terms of energy, frequency and vibration.
Nicolas Tesla

Everything is energy and that is all. Match the frequency of the reality You want and you cannot help but get that reality. It can be no other way. This is not philosophy. This is physics.
Albert Einstein

GLOSSARY

Frequency: Energy has a vibration and the rate a vibration happens creates a wave. Energy can do this in two ways: 1) as sound in the material/matter world or 2) as an electromagnetic field: radio, infrared and gamma rays. Both are measured in seconds called Hertz. When a vibration completes one cycle per second then the frequency is one Hertz. If it completes 432 cycles per second then its 432-Hertz (Hz).

Hertz is named after a German scientist, Rudolf Hertz, who invented how to measure the waves. Because waves are so vast and come is so many different frequencies, especially higher frequencies like electromagnetic ones, we need higher systems of measurement to accommodate them. Some of the ways to measure waves are:

Mega Hertz is 1,000,000 Hertz (for computers)

Giga Hertz is 1,000, 000,000 Hertz. (for computers)

Nano Hertz is one thousand-millionth (10^{9th}) of a hertz. Gamma rays are measured in nano hertz, because the energy frequency is extremely high.

Spectrum, is a band of different colors, such as the colors we can visibly see with our naked eye, that are produced by their different degrees of length of waves (or wavelength). Also includes higher bands of unseen "colors" or wavelengths of energy caused by electromagnetic radiation such as gamma, infrared, x-rays and ultraviolet rays.

Fractal. Fractal comes from the root word that means broken or fractured. A fractal is a never-ending pattern of HOW matter self organizes complex patterns that are self-similar but are different in scale or size in the macro and micro worlds. It is a repeated simple "looping" of the same self similar pattern. Some examples of fractal arrangements are: mountains, clouds, river networks, lightning, broccoli, ferns, trees and their leaves, snow flakes and DNA.

Torus: See glossary in part 3.

TOTAL (known) Spectrum of Wavelength and Frequency

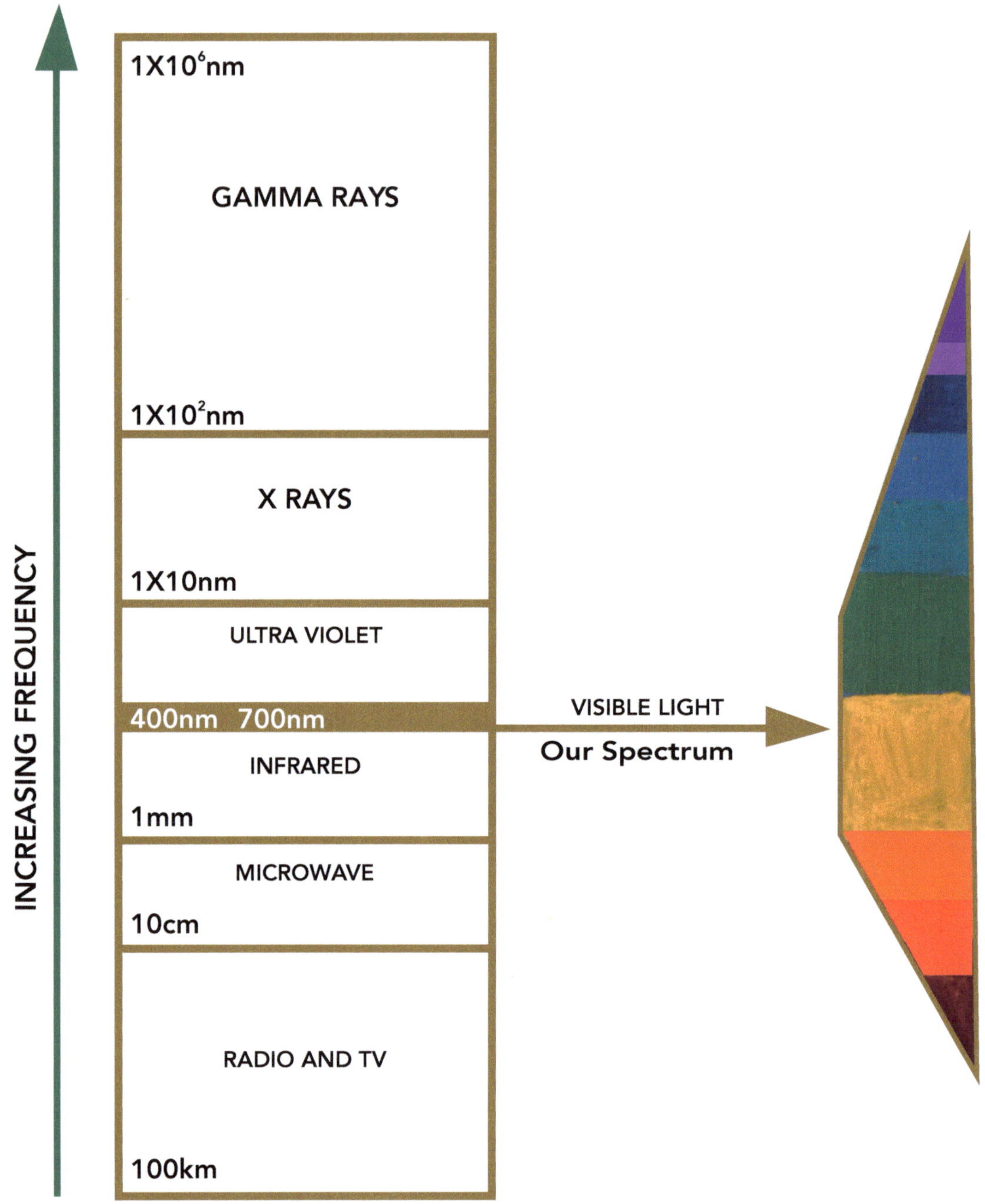

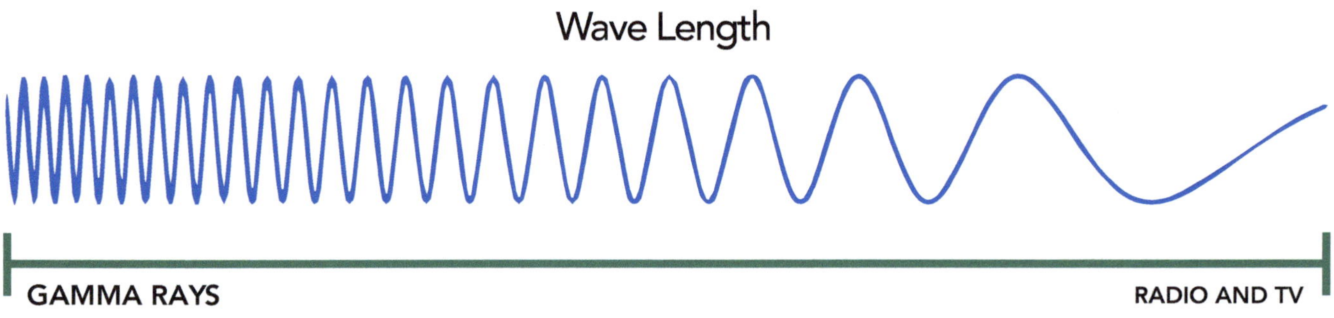

↑ INCREASING FREQUENCY

- 1×10^6 nm
- GAMMA RAYS
- 1×10^2 nm
- X RAYS
- 1×10 nm
- ULTRA VIOLET
- 400nm 700nm → VISIBLE LIGHT / Our Spectrum
- INFRARED
- 1mm
- MICROWAVE
- 10cm
- RADIO AND TV
- 100km

Wave Length

GAMMA RAYS — RADIO AND TV

Frequency, Wave Length and Proton Scales
and their relation to color.

This chart shows: 1. frequency vibration (Hertz), 2. wave length (nm) and 3. proton scales. The scales are approximate between 380 nm and 900 nm. These are the only waves that are visible to the naked eye in our 3D world.

How to read the chart
Frequency rises or increases as you move from right to left.
Wave lengths become longer as you read left to right.

1. Frequency (energy) (hertz, Hz).

Violet	Indigo	Blue	Green	Yellow	Orange	Red	Red-Brown
850-750	675	630	590	525	510	450	380

2. Wave length (nanometers, (nm) the higher the number the tighter the wave length)

| 400 | 445 | 475 | 570 | 590 | 650 | 780 | |

3. Proton energy (in electron volts (eV)

| 3.1 | 2.8 | 2.6 | 2.4 | 2.2 | 2.1 | 1.9 | 1.6 |

Colors, musical scale and their relationship to the emotions.

Color chart scales. On this page we will see how colors, hertz and musical tones correspond to the emotions. The chart starts from full expansion of the higher emotions and descends down to the lower emotions. Independent studies have shown that the DNA strands respond to lower emotions by tightening or constricting their structure. The higher emotions relax the flow of energy and promotes the ability of DNA to self organize, based on the efficient PHI ratio and fractal structure. Note. The range of the Hertz scale used below are approximate.

COLOR	HERTZ	MUSICAL TONE	EMOTION
Violet	850-1000 hertz	SI=B	Enlightenment, perfect state, awakened, compassion
Indigo	750-850 hertz	LA=A	Return to spiritual order, intuition, compassion
Blue	750-750 hertz	SO=G	Understanding, peace, creativity, joy, forgiveness and healing
Green	650-700 hertz	FA=F	Balance, love and connection to self, acceptance
Yellow	525-650 hertz	MI=E	Will power, inner strength, trust, courage, perseverance
Orange	480-525 hertz	RE=D	Pride, anger, desire, blame, hopelessness, fear, jealousy and envy
Red *Rojo*	360-480 hertz	DO=C	Grief, apathy, guilt, shame, hatred, greed and rage.

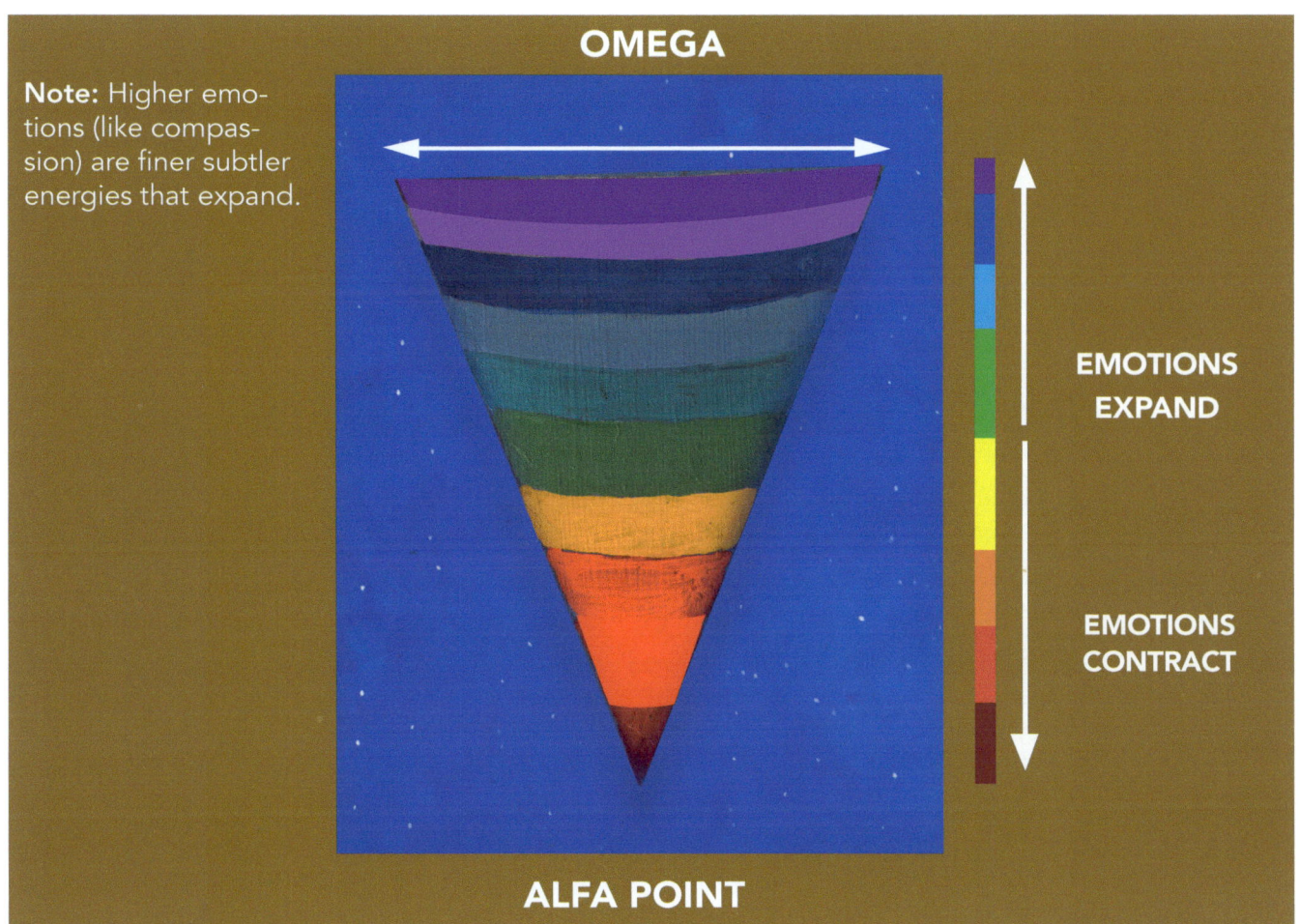

How the emotions work according to this chart. Lower emotions have a longer wave and a lower frequency energy rate (anger). Higher emotions have a shorter wavelength and a higher frequency (compassion). An emotion such as anger has a constricting and tightening affect on the whole body and the mind because it has a lower vibration rate and a longer wavelength. The lower emotions reside in the lowest part of the cone. Constrictive emotions tighten the energy flow within the entire body, which puts stress on the organs, glands and the nervous system. Long term unresolved lower constrictive emotions can cause the organs and other parts of the body to malfunction and in some cases cause serious illness and even death. The lower emotions also overwork the adrenal glands because they keep the body in a constant state of anxiousness, excitement and/or stress. One can use the mid-level and higher emotions to help overcome the lower emotions. As one reflects and searches for the reasons behind the anger (as an example) and notices when it arises and makes an effort to avoid those situations, and/or matures and/or finds an answer to deal with the anger, they are then on their way to resolving and healing. They will discover that the mid range emotions such as courage, perseverance and inner strength can be used to overcome such lower emotions. As we use the higher emotions, such as compassion, we begin to expand even higher into the upper cone. When resolving lower emotions, one will notice that the actual anger (as in this case) wasn't destroyed, or stuffed or ignored; the emotions evolved. It was dealt with by using the mid range to higher heart emotions in combination with a more conscious, disciplined and awake mind.

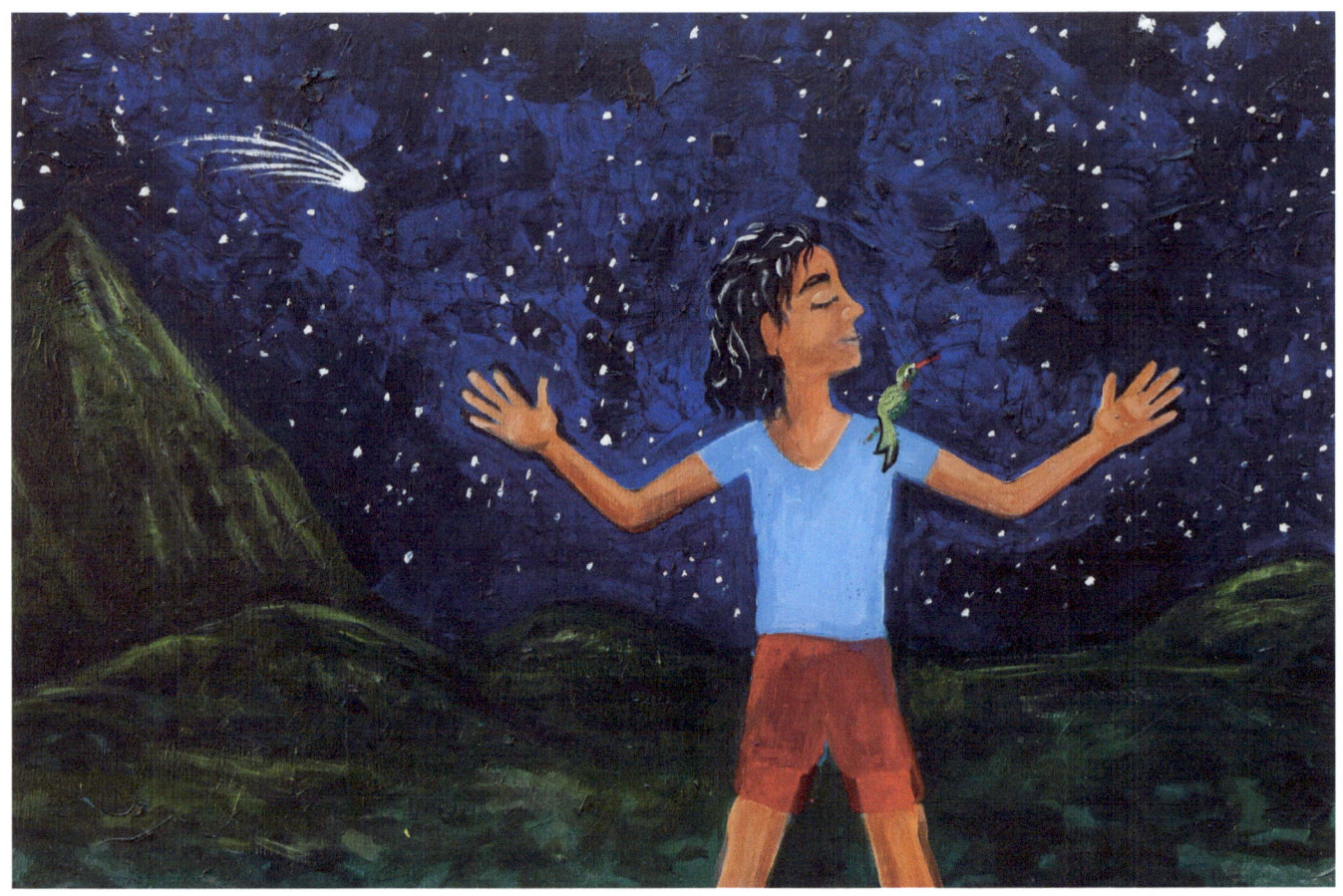

In the following example Matisse combines his self-analysis (mind) and his mid to high range emotions to overcome a lower emotion such as anger. Matisse notices that every time he has to read aloud in class he gets nervous and then gets angry. Matisse decides to investigate WHY he has such a connection between: reading aloud, nervousness and anger. He makes a decision to find his own answers to resolve this association and connection. He then sits and meditates for a while and comes up with several options and a plan. Matisse just empowered himself by choosing to resolve his own problem by using these mid-range emotions: will power, perseverance and courage.

Matisse realizes that he could use some help so he explains to his teacher his situation and asks if he could skip reading aloud for a week. He also asks his best friend Lucy for help. (SeeMore is proud that Matisse is figuring out how to resolve his own problems). Lucy then explains that the class is not "laughing" at him for the reasons he thinks, which is that he is a bad reader. Lucy informs him that they are not laughing but are amused because they like how he says some of his words because of his accent. They actually look forward to him reading because they want to imitate his accent. Matisse is relieved to hear such news and realizes how he thought something completely different. With this realization, he feels relieved and notes his anger is going away. This new information begins the association and disconnection of certain emotions with reading aloud that caused the stress, which led to anger. Matisse analyzed his situation again and considered the new information that included his accent. Matisse decided he liked his accent but that he also wanted to pronounce certain words more accurately and worked on that. Matisse used his newly found solutions and when it was his turn to read aloud he was less nervous and less stressed, which in the past caused him to get angry. This time his anger didn't surface so much because he had empowered himself with knowledge of his situation. Thanks to Lucy, his teacher and Matisse's own ability and maturity for assuming his responsibility in resolving his own problems, Matisse empowered himself. He exercised his abilities by using these higher mid-range emotions: will power, perseverance and courage. He was able to connect these to self by choosing to heal. Matisse also realized that by forgiving himself (for not acting and believing in himself sooner) he could also forgive his classmates. He realized they also suffer from their own misinterpretations about themselves and others. This realization then caused Matisse to experience compassion, one of the most evolved of all the emotions, not only for himself but also for his classmates.

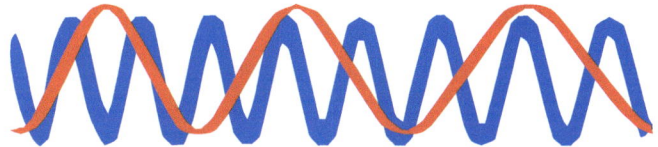

Lower emotions have long waves (red). Higher emotions have shorter waves (blue). The lower emotions are canceled out by higher frecuency waves. Matisse used his mid-range and higher emotions to overcome the lower emotions.

Spiritual Tool: How to by-pass the lower emotions when struggling to transmute their frequencies.

Sometimes we become frustrated by our lack of progress to manage and overcome our lower emotions. Our higher emotions are developing but they are battling with the other side of ourselves that is still entangled with our lower emotions.
There is a way to bypass this struggle temporarily by reaching in and connecting with our higher Self, the Self that is connected to the Soul. Through prayer and strong intention we can request direct communication and connection with our Soul. The Soul will respond in a variety of ways including dreams, insights, synchonicities and/or "coincidences". The Soul will always respond to our authentic pleas of the higher emotions: understanding, forgiveness, appreciation, valor, and/or compassion. We can also use this same method when we are experiencing difficulty in communicating with a significant other (living or deceased) that is in our life or a part of our life. WE do this first by contacting our own inner higher Self and asking It to contact the higher Self of the significant other (mom, dad, brother, teacher, friend and/or perceived "enemy").
One's higher Self will first ask for permission on your behalf, to engage in open communication the other's higher Self. The intent must be pure and for the higher good of each and for others (family and community). When the higher Selves engage, the usual games, defenses and/or other lower ego emotions are by-passed or are over-ridden by the pureness of intent and by the Soul's inability to engage in lower emotions. Clues and/or realizations are then presented and revealed to both sides corresponding to the uniqueness and individuality of each personality. In other words, the higher Self knows exactly HOW to say and WHAT information you need precisely. This will enable you, in this moment, to overcome the block within yourself and loosen and manifest a path toward resolution.

The Soul will always accept an opportunity to aide one in their quest in "knowing thyself". This translates into meeting the challenges that life presents to us, through relationships. The relationships in its joy and challenges provide opportunities for us to emotionally and spirituality mature. Our relationships with others will change and evolve as we individually change and evolve.

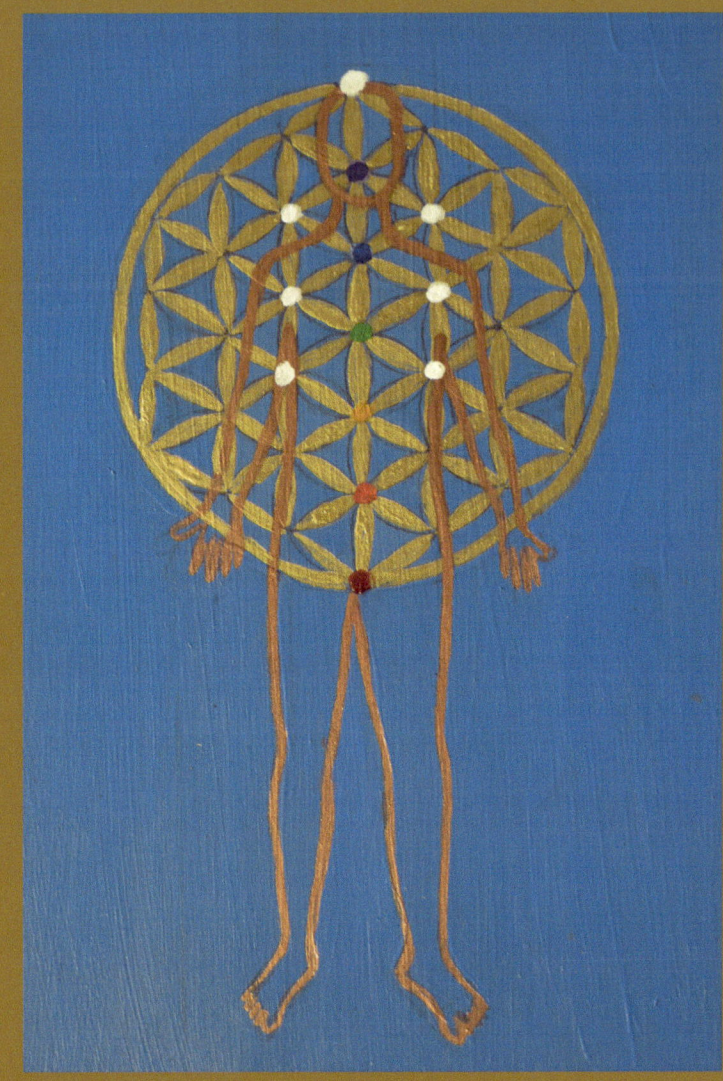

Part 5. Ancient Schools of Wisdom
Kabbalah and the 13 Sephiroth
The Three Pillars of Life
Inverted Tree of Life

Cabal comes from the word Kabbalah, a 16th century word (but much older) which was/ is a part of the Jewish and Agnostic chakra system traditions. However in recent history it has come to signify "a small group of secret plotters as against a government or person in authority." There are other negative definitions. In this book we use the original meaning of the word, which signifies a religious/spiritual chakra system that was originally intended to unite and connect man to Creator and the Divine. Over the centuries and most profoundly in our recent history, this word has become contrary; its divinity has been eliminated and perverted from its original version. This casts a horrible shadow on spiritual wisdom that the Kabbalah offers. Its practices and insights can potentially assist one in creating their own respective *map* that can lead one back to their own Divinity, which is one´s reconnection to God/First Source.

SEPHIROTH OF THE KABBALAH

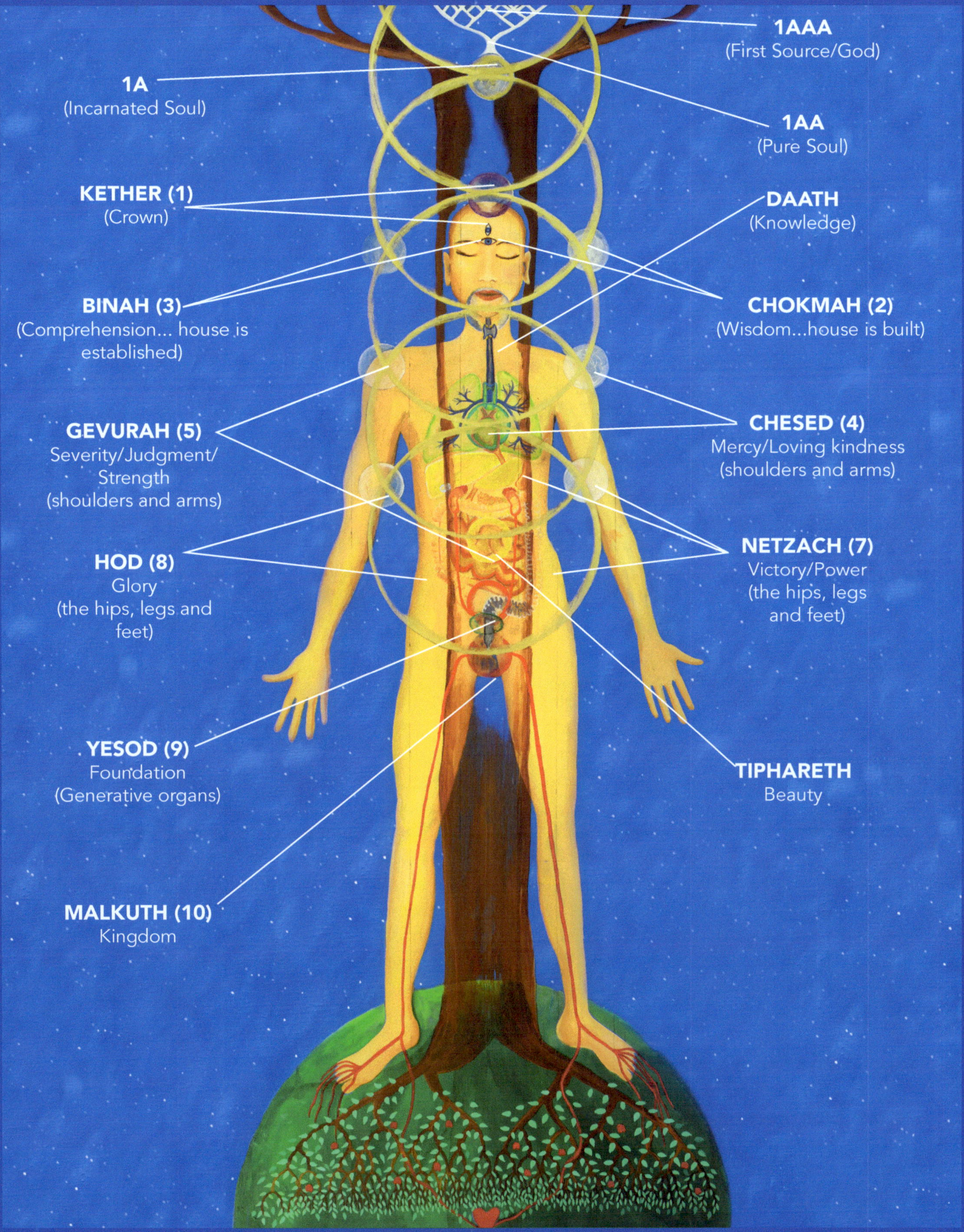

1AAA
(First Source/God)

1A
(Incarnated Soul)

1AA
(Pure Soul)

KETHER (1)
(Crown)

DAATH
(Knowledge)

BINAH (3)
(Comprehension... house is established)

CHOKMAH (2)
(Wisdom...house is built)

GEVURAH (5)
Severity/Judgment/
Strength
(shoulders and arms)

CHESED (4)
Mercy/Loving kindness
(shoulders and arms)

HOD (8)
Glory
(the hips, legs and feet)

NETZACH (7)
Victory/Power
(the hips, legs and feet)

YESOD (9)
Foundation
(Generative organs)

TIPHARETH
Beauty

MALKUTH (10)
Kingdom

GLOSSARY AND HISTORICAL BACKROUND

Kabbalah (cabbala or cabala or Cabbalah). Webster dictionary definition: "A medieval and modern system of Jewish theosophy, mysticism and thaumaturgy (performance of miracles and/ or magic) marked by the belief in creation through emanation and a cipher (coded) method of interpreting Scripture." Note: We will use this definition as a base. We will also attempt to give a more complete definition and expand on its implied significance in this section of the book.

Sephiroth or Sefirot or Sephirot are plural. Selfirah or Sephirah is singular.
There are 10 Sephiroth and some believe there are 11 Sephiroth *jewels* that can guide our interior towards our real being or divine being. The Jewish and Agnostic traditions believe in these basic 10 (Jewish) or 11 (Agnostic) Sephiroth.

In this book we will condense the information of each Sephiroth and give an overview of the Kabbalah and each of the 13 Sephiroth based on some of the studies of Master Choa Kok Sui from his book, *The Spiritual Essence*. The Works of Parmahansa Yogananda, Sri Ramana Maharshi as well as other great masters and the ancient Tibetan Buddhism studies are also included in this interpretation. All these sacred works share similar quests and disciplines in the search for the same thing: illumination or self-realization or cosmic consciousness. An attempt will also be made to include the Kabbalah's relationship to the Three Pillars of Life and the Inverted Tree of Life. The Kabbalah, as with all great spiritual texts, requires great study and devotion to unlock, understand and adopt its *jewels* or keys. These are the keys that help liberate one´s soul from the material world and its ties to reincarnation or *recycling*. This is just an overview to help expose the grandeur of these *sacred* works historically shrouded in secrecy and half-truths.

Kabbalah is an ancient mystical "occult" (secret) tradition based on the Sephiroth.
There are 13 Sephiroth and they are creative forces or *jewels* that can intervene on the *behalf* of one who learns, practices and becomes the teaching of each Selfirah. The Sephiroth intervene on behalf of man, who lives in the material world of form, and God/Infinite/First Source/Creator.

The Sephiroth physical positions are based on the Three Pillars of Life (similar to the positions of Platonic Solids and Metraton´s Cube). However, Master Choa Kok Sui believes that the ancients may not have realized that the left side of the brain controls the right side of the body and the right side of the brain controls the left side of the body. The Pillars of Life are therefore switched and are contrary from the Jewish and Agnostic Traditions. Here it will be reversed: the left side of the brain controls right side of the body, so the right side will correspond to the Pillar of Severity; the right side of the brain controls the left side of the body so it will correspond to the Pillar of Mercy.

Kabbalah and Sephiroth explained.
It appears that the Sephiroth are activated by authenticity, practice and a strong desire to connect, merge and/or BE one with First Source or God. As the energy wheel or chakra or Sephiroth become more activated to the point that one's energy is healthy, one then evolves to the next step, which is to transform or transmute that energy and move up it to the next higher chakra wheel and awaken it. Each step along the spine and it's the corresponding chakra wheel, increases one's experiences in unity and equanimity, leading towards liberation from the realm of extreme duality.

This probability increases exponentially when one uses multiple Sephiroth simultaneously as they reinforce, accentuate and are interdependent on each other. This is intelligence in motion that creates balance and harmony. It appears, that as the energy in the chakras changes and rises, it also expands. This action causes a change in frequency, allowing one to become more aligned with the Infinite Creator or God. As one continues to connect and practice, one will begin to resonate more and more with that higher frequency, discarding old ways, habits and desires of the material world. The Kabbalah, it appears, can serve as a *passport* into the higher realms. It also appears that as we evolve individually and collectively we can potentially change everything, including the matrix, along the way! This could mean that if we were to practice the jewels we would be empowered enough to connect our Self to the Divine. It then appears that we each are *the secret*, because we each have the keys to unlock our own potential. Our potential relies on our ability to authentically remember who we are and that responsibility is our own. The only thing that really separates us from each other is WHEN we each decide to make this empowering journey.

Other important facts, history and connections to the Kabbalah and the Sephiroth. It appears that there is a deep mystery and secrecy surrounding the Kabbalah. The Jewish Tradition has kept the Kabbalah alive for many centuries and it can be dated back to the Old Testament. It appears that the Jewish tradition has guarded and not revealed all that the Kabbalah is. Also there is evidence that the Kabbalah goes back even further than the Old Testament, mainly because of its association with one of the most ancient of all symbols, the Flower of Life. In fact, the Kabbalah fits neatly within that Flower of Life form. I believe that many cultures have/had similar *secret* associations respectively, that are/were equally as empowering. But in our collective planetary history, that information gets lost, burned (The Great Library of Alexandra by the Romans) or stolen or locked away (the Vatican). So historically, these keys were hidden and became secret and known only to a few. It follows that our individual, as well as our collective *passports* have become postponed or canceled. The path or a Path has been side tracked by half-truths or lies or worse buried or destroyed. This leaves the rest of us blind and ignorant, never knowing that we each are *the key* and that we are already connected. These jewels are the knowledge of the Sephiroth and they are sacred and knowing of them (or some similar knowledge) empowers the Self, liberating one from a life of seemingly endless reincarnations, or what I like to more accurately refer to as the recycling of the soul. These jewels are keys that can turn on and drive the great energy engine Sephiroth of You, all we need do is claim those keys and use them. It basically appears that the Sephiroth are a plea to invite the Divine or God to live and dwell within us as US, each individually. In other words, the Divine dwells within you as YOU... as we awaken, we see and realize this more and more.

Prana is a Hindu word/concept that means life force or lifetrons. It is finer than atomic energy. It is potential creation and it permeates the cosmos and anything that has life in it.

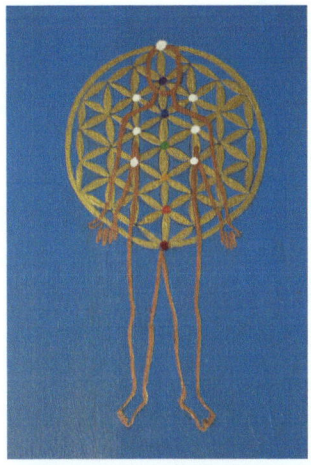

Figure 1. The human form and the Flower of Life fit perfectly on the points (nodes) in the Kabbalah (chakras).

Kabbalah and the 13 Sephiroth
(For your consideration)

Preface. The two top chakras or Sephiroth, are located over the top of the head, over the crown chakra, Kether. These two chakras have been totally eliminated, ignored and/or are virtually non-existent in our worldview. Few writings exist connecting the higher realms to the human being form, in which the soul ONLY temporarily resides. In order for us to even exist, thought always precedes matter or form. Physics also validates that form is always preceded by thought and ideas. The fact that many life forms share the same *blueprint* based on the same mathematical PHI expressions whether its one-dimensional or 2D or 3D form shows thought preceded those form (s). Another fact is humans have systems that are highly complex and involve an aspect of *self* or a consciousness of self. This self consciousness seems to have a life that is separate and independent of a physical body self. Also, the fact that we use only 10 to 20% of our brain capacity and that 90% of our DNA is inactive are two facts about the human condition that are suspicious. This information has far reaching implications and speculations about who or what "creator" could activate or inactivate portions of DNA in a species? It would be a different story if it wasn´t manifested but it is... where is the other 90%? This means most of who we are is asleep and we are not accessing the larger portions of our brains and DNA. Also that some scientists label the other 90% of that inactive DNA as *junk* also makes it more probable that something is being hidden. In fact, all of these reasons motivate me to be very suspicious and more importantly inquisitive. Therefore, (in this section of the book) the Root or Source, is reconnected to ITS creation, the human form.

The Divine and ITS Cord of Light and the journey into Matter: 1AAA

THE SOURCE of EVERYTHING and ITS connection is forever maintained with and to everything. God or First Source is the "Ocean" of everything.

Second Sephirah above Kether: 1AA

Part of the Ocean decides to become a "drop" or soul. The *drop* separates and decides to descend into the material world. As the soul descends into matter, it forgets more and more of its connection to Source or God but the soul is and will always be connected. The "drop of Ocean" soul maintains its connection always through the ROOT of the Source of All or OCEAN of ALL, no matter how far it descends. The Root is the Divine connection for the soul, without it the soul would cease its individual *drop* existence.

Sephirah right above Kether (the Crown Chakra) is the Incarnated Soul: 1A

According to the Inverted Tree of Life, the spiritual root descends down further into the incarnated soul zone. The cord of light travels down from the drop of pure soul and connects and supplies the templates or blueprints to the etheric zones of the spiritual, emotional and mental bodies of You. It is located at the upper perimeter of our auric field over the top of the head and continues around all of the body, encasing it. These outer fields help construct the human form with a *body blueprint* that is used for the actual body. The blueprint of the body and the actual body occupy the same space (or ether); this is why special cameras can detect limbs that are non existing after amputations or accidents. This incarnated soul is separate BUT connected always through the root, as the divine energy descends and lives or resides in ethereal forms of you descending in its final destination of the physical form. When you *re-awaken* you will begin the journey back to Source/Creator. Until ascension, you are a human form *container*, with a PHI based structure, living in the 3D material world (hologram) of matter or form, subject to the laws of nature and physics.

The journey back. As one spiritually progresses and *remembers*, the Root cord becomes thicker, wider and stronger…it is our direct access to the Divine and all that is, was and will BE. Spiritual evolution consists of authentically actualizing coherence between body, mind, emotions, soul and actions; only this can re-strengthen the "forgotten" Root cord, the bond between the drop of ocean (the Soul) and The Source, (The Ocean of All).

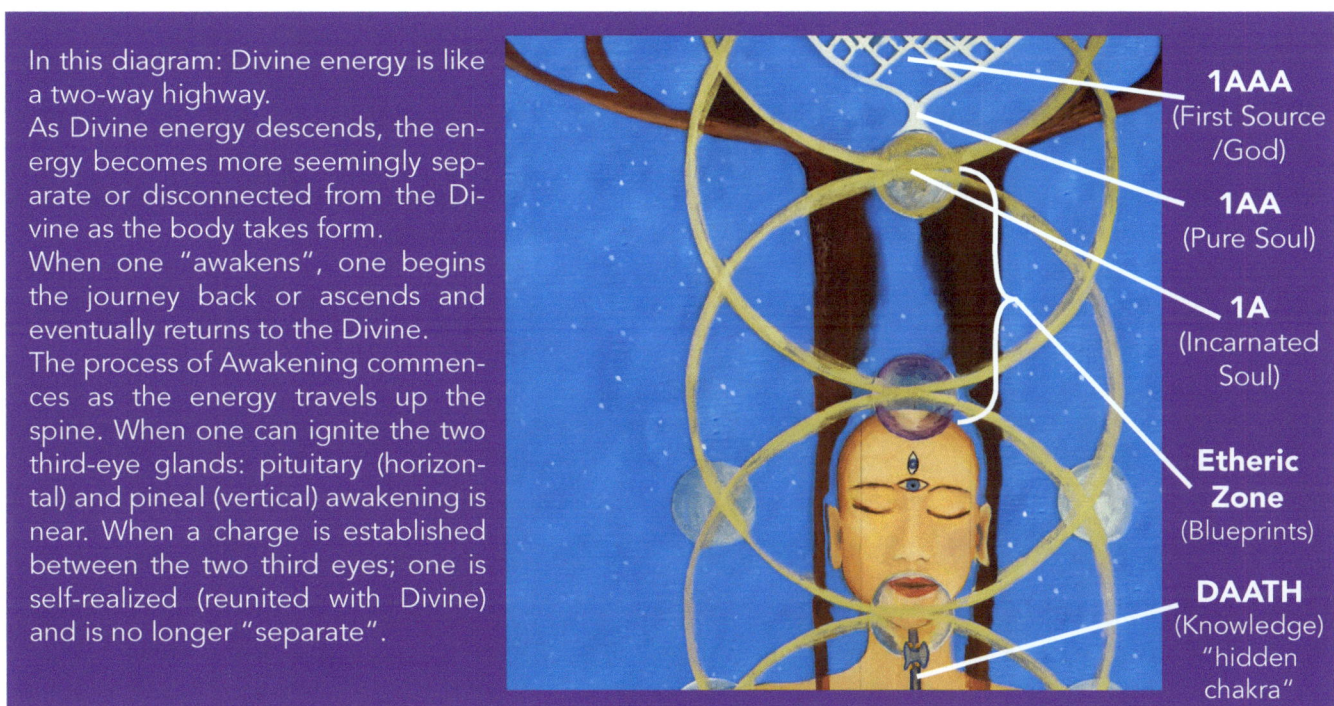

In this diagram: Divine energy is like a two-way highway.
As Divine energy descends, the energy becomes more seemingly separate or disconnected from the Divine as the body takes form.
When one "awakens", one begins the journey back or ascends and eventually returns to the Divine.
The process of Awakening commences as the energy travels up the spine. When one can ignite the two third-eye glands: pituitary (horizontal) and pineal (vertical) awakening is near. When a charge is established between the two third eyes; one is self-realized (reunited with Divine) and is no longer "separate".

1AAA (First Source /God)
1AA (Pure Soul)
1A (Incarnated Soul)
Etheric Zone (Blueprints)
DAATH (Knowledge) "hidden chakra"

11 DAATH in the Kabbalah means knowledge. Daath is the hidden abyss center or chakra. It is the center of concrete mental faculty or knowledge acquisition. It controls and energizes the throat, larynx, trachea, thyroid, parathyroid and lymphatic (immune) system. Daath is connected to the throat chakra, the center for higher creativity and Daath is also connected to the sacral sex chakra, the center of procreation or lower creativity. Daath and the sex chakra (Yesod) work in tandem. Having a healthy sex chakra is mandatory in transmuting energy. One cannot evolve without it; it's the fundamental building block that nourishes the higher chakras. As the energy ascends to the subtler realms where the higher emotions are located in the higher chakras, the energy frequency there is much higher and intense. The sex chakra provides this additional needed energy and it becomes the source of sustenance and empowerment for one's spiritual evolution.

Daath also is referred to as the abyss of the incarnated soul that was and is separated from its pure soul, the part that descended and incarnated into form. It is referred to as the abyss because we forget and become *lost* in our increasing attachments to our self, the senses, knowledge acquisition and the material world in which we live. (OR) We can exercise our choice by re-membering or re-uniting through (yoga). We can re-connect the higher soul with the incarnated soul… through activation of all chakras in harmony and ascending back up (3,2 and 1 and above) to higher soul. DAATH is no longer the abyss but becomes the *bridge*, to remembering and reuniting with SOURCE.

Note about "Kosher": What comes out of the mouth is more important than what goes in, as referenced by the word *kosher* which means pure or clean. It is of greater importance to practice *kosher* thoughts, *kosher* speech and *kosher* actions rather than putting importance on consuming kosher foods.

Note: "With Wisdom (Chokmah) a house is built, with Understanding (Binah) it is established, and with Knowledge (Daath) the rooms are filled." Proverbs 24: 3-4. All chakras below Daath are tied to the incarnated soul.
Credit: Master Choa Kok Sui

SEPHIROTH 1-10:
Refer to Kabbalah/Sephiroth diagram at the beginning of this section.
These Sephiroth are from the Jewish and Agnostic traditions (similar to Hindu and Buddhist traditions).

1 KETHER SEPHIRAH. The Kether Sephirah is located on the crown of the head and it is the center of Oneness. It is the inverted tree's root point of entry into matter or form. Kether is the third eye placed vertically.

The root's point of entry of divine energy into human form is the pineal gland. Higher soul is incarnated and the body is *manifested*. The pineal gland is the direct knowing terminal to higher soul, but it is NOT the higher soul. Higher intuition is direct knowing. Direct knowing is like taking your computer (pineal gland) USB cord and plugging it into the Mother Computer or cosmic consciousness, on a need to know basis. Your USB cord is plugged into the center of spiritual consciousness or divine oneness or cosmic consciousness. It is where full expansion is illuminated because one has self realized while in the material body form. It is: "I am that I am", there is no separation. Everything is connected because you are *plugged in* and have instant access whenever you need answers and/or guidance or when there is a desire *to be* with the Divine.

2 CHOKMAH SEPHIRAH. Chokmah means wisdom in the Kabbalah. This is the center of wisdom and lower intuition. Chokmah is the third eye between the eyebrows placed horizontally and it is also ruled by the pineal gland. In Chokmah, the pineal gland is more connected to the body through the pituitary/master gland, as opposed to Kether where it is more connected to cosmic consciousness or *Mother Computer*.

This third eye chakra energizes and controls the pineal gland and the nervous system, where the Root further descends into the spine. It also controls the right side of the brain, which controls left side of the body. Lower Buddha or lower intuition (not cosmic consciousness) is to know through seeing with the inner eye of the pineal gland. It is inner perception without having to use logic or reason. It is clairvoyance through visions and hearing, but not direct knowing like Kether.

3 BINAH SEPHIRAH. Binah in the Kabbalah means understanding. This is the center of understanding, higher mental abstract abilities and the alignment of will to Source. It is the third eye, between eyebrows ruled by pituitary gland. This chakra also controls and energizes the pituitary gland. The pituitary gland is the master gland so it directly and indirectly affects all other systems and organs of the body. It is the center of intelligent will, which precedes intelligent action. Intelligence is not to be confused with the acquisition of knowledge just for itself, which is sterile. Intelligent will and action are both necessary; together they produce results by becoming intelligence in motion. Intelligent will is also important because it is the ability to express the abstract, the concept and/or the principle; to put into words the highest wisdom and making the *word* or intelligence available to others.

Note: Chokmah and Binah work hand in hand or in tandem especially when the spark or charge is ignited between the pineal and pituitary glands. This charge creates access to the Divine, strengthening the Root (that descended into form) to return to the Divine (ascension or reuniting with God).

4 CHESED SEPHIRAH. Chesed means mercy and loving kindness in the Kabbalah. The heart chakra (front and back) is the center of the emotional heart and self will power.
The front of the heart controls and energizes the heart and thymus gland. The back of the heart relates to prana or lifetron flow, affects the circulatory system, lungs and thymus gland (defender of the body). CHESED is the center for higher emotions: peace, compassion, joy, gentleness, caring, patience etc. When the heart chakra is as equally developed as the solar plexus chakra, there is a balance of self love and love of others. There is also a balance between the material and spiritual aspects of life. Love of self must come first, then it connects to the Kether Sephirah, the chakra of love for all that is or universal love. "You must see your Self as worthy before you see another as worthy. You must see your Self as blessed before you can see another as blessed. You must first know your Self to be holy before you can acknowledge the holiness in another". The Heart also contains the physical Soul Seed. This seed is what gives life to the physical form. The seed leaves when physical death occurs. Quote credit: Master Choa Kok Sui.

5 GEVURAH SEPHIRAH. Gevurah in the Kabbalah means severity, judgment and strength. It is the center of the following: 1. lower/higher emotions: justice, strength, perseverance, fairness and courage and 2. the center of negative lower emotions: anger, hatred, destructiveness, worry, tension, aggressiveness, addiction and criticalness. The solar plexus chakra (front and back of body) is also the center of emotion and will. Gevurah chakra controls and energizes diaphragm, pancreas, liver and stomach. It also energizes the "psychology" of the large and small intestine, appendix, lungs, heart and all parts of the body. Over-activation of the lower emotions directly and adversely affects the lower chakras, creating a vicious cycle that continuously refuels it self. Gevuruh is where the lower will is located and it is also where the will of the masses is located. When one makes the decision to separate one's will from the will of the masses, they become aligned with and have more access to using the higher (lower) emotions of the Gevuruh chakra. Access to these higher lower emotions of this chakra are the foundation emotions that give strength to the evolutionary process that progresses into the expansion or flowering of the higher emotions located in the chakras of the heart and above. The act to separate one's will is actually intelligence in action or motion and it commences a crucial crossroad in one's spiritual evolution. This change of will solidifies that a unique journey within has started and that intelligent action is officially and authentically activated. This is the only way it can be activated, it's the commencement of a one-on-one relationship with the Divine. This is where First Source/God /Cosmic Consciousness can speak and guide one directly.

Note: Chesed (4) represents and controls left shoulder and left arm. And Gevuruh (5) represents and controls right shoulder and right arm. Arms are used to embrace with love meant for ALL (4) or attack in fear or anger (5) (and most people are right handed). Cheped (love and mercy) and Gevuruh (severity and justice) need to be balanced; they are polar opposites. "Too much severity and justice becomes cruel and too much mercy and love in the form of tolerance creates chaos. Gevuruh in its extreme manifests as a police or totalitarian state where there is fear and lack of freedom. This type of justice must be balanced with Chesed where justice is transformative and therapeutic. Lawmakers and politicians must realize that the breaking of laws are usually caused by stressed and psychologically ill cultures that keep their citizens tied to an unjust system where their lives and means of living have been reduced to mere or non-existent survival levels". Quote credit: Master Choa Kok Sui.

Note: The top five Sephirah opposites are as follows: Kether's virtue is good will; its opposite is maliciousness and ruthlessness. Chokmah's virtue is wisdom; its opposite is foolishness. Binah and Daath virtues are truth; its opposite is to lie. Cheped's virtues are love and kindness and its opposite is hatred. Gevuruh's virtue is justice and its opposite is injustice. Credit: Master Choa Kok Sui.

6 TIPHARETH SEPHIRAH. Tiphareth means beauty in the Kabbalah; this is the center for instinct in knowing. It is located in the navel chakra, which controls and energizes the small and large intestines and appendix. It also controls and regulates the base Sephirah Malkuth, center of actions. This is the center of CHI and is not to be confused with prana, which is life force energy. CHI has to do with all forms of energy: 1. food, the quality of it is directly linked to its vitality, which graciously comes from the Earth 2. one's vitality from one's environment (emotionally supportive or destructive) 3. one's vitality in the commitment to serving life (efforts made to reconnect within one's self spiritually in service to self and others). 4. one's vitality and growing ability to connect in love and intutive knowing. 5. and lastly, one's ability to disconnect from the senses in meditation in order to restore and connect within Self and to the Divine. All of these along *with* prana (the quantity of and the quality of) affects one's prana or life force. This is what makes you alive and drives You; it is your CHI, all energies combined (one-five). What you think, do and also your intent influences the overall vitalness and quality of CHI. Connecting with one's CHI and strengthening it and the body allows for better flow and overall health. One's CHI is the *divine vault* to everything and most importantly to one's spiritual evolution.

Note: "Good thoughts correspond to Binah Sephirah. Good heart corresponds to Daath, the throat chakra. Good will to the solar plexus chakra. Good actions correponds to the Gevurah Sephirah of the navel chakra. The Tiphareth Sephirah is a combination of all of these chakras: good thoughts, good words, good heart and good will manifest good actions on Earth". In other words, this is how we create *on Earth as it is in Heaven.* Quote credit: Master Choa Kok Sui.

7 NETZACH SEPHIRAH. Netzach means victory and power in the Kabbalah. Its center is in the spleen, the source of power and life energy (prana). Netzach directly affects our actual sense of success and victory. The spleen converts and distributes white prana (original life force) into all colors for all the chakras in the body. The spleen chakra, front and back of body have the same functions as the physical spleen that acts as a filter to purify the blood, which also enhances the immune system. It purifies the blood by recycling healthy red blood cells and discarding unusable and damaged ones. It is also the place where white blood cells, which produce antibodies that destroy pathogens, are stored. The spleen chakra has two other responsibilities: it directly energizes and controls the physical spleen and it affects the amount, quality and distribution of prana throughout the body. The spleen's success affects the over all health (victory) of the body. Netzach chakra is closely related to the navel chakra and they can work together optimizing each other's functions by healing, purifying and increasing each other's energy flow. The importance or *victory* of a highly functioning spleen not only filters and purifies the blood, but can additionally 1) contribute to the amount of prana able to enter the body and 2) distribute that prana to all parts of the body including the etheric fields. The spleen´s victory can be greatly increase by meditation, self mastery of the lower negative emotions and by practicing healthier ways and diets that do not over work the spleen. This can be accomplished by periods of rest and fasting where the spleen can use its energy increasing and distributing prana more efficiently throughout the body.

Chakras 6 and 7 function together and regulate each other.

8 HOD SEPHIRAH. Hod means glory in the Kabbalah. This center is ruled by the Meng Mein (means "gate of life" in Chinese) chakra and it controls and energizes the kidneys, adrenal glands and blood pressure. It is located in back of the navel. The Hod chakra serves as a pumping station or elevator at lower spine and moves the prana energy upward into the higher chakras. Hod has the power to transmute lower (lead) energy to golden energy. There are three important alchemical centers corresponding to the three physical zones of the human body where Hod or glory can be transmuted from lead to gold. The first is the Meng Mein chakra, it is the *etheric alchemical* center where Hod can transmute into glory. The second one is the back heart chakra, it is the *emotional alchemical* center where the emotions can transmute into Hod or glory. The third one is the crown chakra, it is the *spiritual alchemical* center where the spiritual energies can transmute into Hod or glory. This is the true meaning and secret of inner alchemy. This transmutation starts with self, proceeds and expands out to include family, communities and nations. One of the most important emotions of this chakra is forgiveness. The act of forgiving encourages both physical and inner healing. The act of forgiving one´s self for our own mistakes paves the way for us to forgive others for theirs.

Glory also means balancing Netzach and Hod. Transforming and transmuting our lower energies on a personal level enables one to also do so on a communal level. When many individuals align themselves and establish a peace within, there is a higher probability and potential to establish peace within communities; from communities to nations. Peace within, creates more options to resolve problems. This is especially useful when potentially volatile situations arise. Peace and authentic communication established within, increases the potential for practicing understanding and compassion; important higher emotions that can help resolve any problem or conflict. Learning to negotiate, compromise, as well as practicing forgiveness are ways that intelligence in motion can manifest: within self, within community, within nation and between nations. The other option as Gandhi said is, "An eye for an eye will leave the whole world blind". Sephiroth 7 Netzach and 8 Hod function and regulate each other. They are the third pair of complimentary opposites that involve the health, balance and transmutation of the energies between victory and power (7) with glory (8). Credit: Master Choa Kok Sui.

Note: Netzach (7) left leg and hip and Hod (8) right leg and hip; hips and legs correspond to energetic, physical and ethereal support for the upper part of the body.

9 YESOD SEPHIRAH. Yesod means foundation in the Kabbalah. Sacred sex chakra controls and energizes the reproductive organs in the pubic area of the human form. Yesod controls and energizes the ovaries in female and testes and prostate glands in males. It also controls and energizes the urethra, bladder, legs and feet for both males and females. This Sephirah is closely connected to (11) DAATH, the throat, chakra of higher creativity. They are strongly linked energetically and operate in tandem. Transmuted sexual energy is paramount in one's spiritual evolution. Therefore one's thoughts, words and actions about the human form (male and female) and sexual relating and relationships need to be addressed and resolved to allow prana and kundalini energies to rise to awaken and transform into the higher chakras. Only a healthy attitude towards sex and its energy can rise to transform and awaken all of the upper chakras into love and spiritual energy. *Healthy* may be viewed as: physical union is a natural act that involves mutual love, respect, and recognition of the divinity within self and one's partner. This is a brief description of an ideal state of being. When the proximity of this state is reached and or strived for, some individuals will make the conscious decision to explore more of their spiritual nature. They will consciously make the decision to transform their procreative (making love) energies into higher creativity energies for their spiritual development. In contrast, an unhealthy view towards sex does not transmute nor does it allow the energy to rise into the upper chakras. When this happens one risks adopting addictive and aggressive behaviors that can become trapped and recycled in the lower chakras. The *first pair of complimentary polar opposites* are Kether and Yesod representing the health, balance and transmutation of the spiritual and sexual energies.

10 MALKUTH SEPHIRAH. Malkuth means kingdom in the Kabbalah. It is the base chakra located in back at the base of spine or coccyx area. The legs and feet are extensions of the base chakra. Self-preservation and instinct for survival that directly involves the adrenal glands are also part of the base chakra. One's ability to work and career choice, the success or lack of, is also associated with the base chakra. This chakra energizes the bone marrow, blood, muscles (the heart being a main one) and skeletal systems hence the whole body. The base chakra is a root taking hold in one's *foundation*; a healthy one produces a strong tree trunk and a weak one the opposite. Kundalini energy (also part of your CHI) is coiled primal cosmic energy (Mother) located

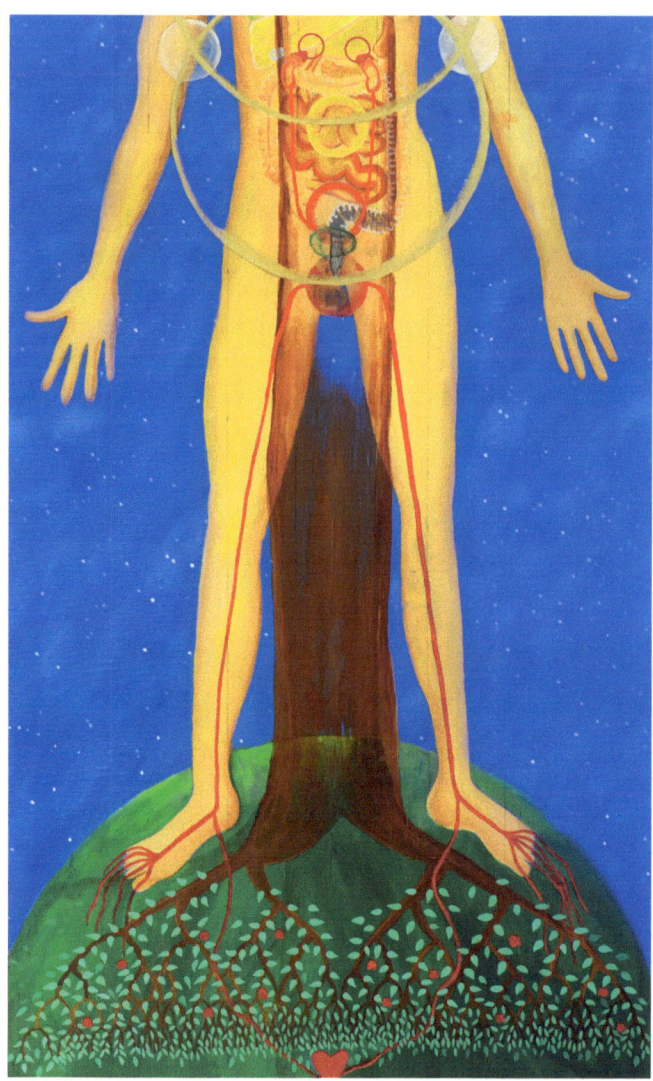

Figure 1. Base chakra includes lower spine, legs, feet and adrenal glands.

at the base of the spine. Many people are unaware that they have this type of energy, which has been represented by ancient civilizations as the coiled serpent. When it is awakened, it travels up the spine awakening good and bad traits alike. This is principally where one's spiritual work and challenges reside. *The second polar opposite* of Malkuth is KETHER. These complimentary polar alchemical opposites involve the importance of health, balance and transmutation of one's spiritual and material worlds. This is accomplished by the kundalini in the spine ascending, while at the same time allowing the Divine or Holy Spirit to descend into the spine. This action is related to the following interpretation, "Heaven on Earth": Heaven, which is Divine… on Earth, which is divine *man*ifestation. Each person, on their respective and unique path, manifests, claims and seizes the responsibilities for their own thoughts, words and actions. Our words, thoughts and actions are our *manifested tree* that we energetically produce and contribute to the Earth. Some will have healthy trees that are strong and can provide and produce fruits and other will contribute in other ways by providing shade, etc. We, the children, can jointly create, through right actions, *Heaven*, by spiritualizing the material world with our uniquely awakened and evolved self that can embrace the Mother and the Father. When the kundalini (primal/Mother/magnetic energy) and prana (life force/breath/Father/electric) energy and our own unique CHI energies are all connected and operating within Self and within many people respectively, then this will be reflected and manifested outward, in the world… as Heaven!

THE 3 PILLARS OF LIFE

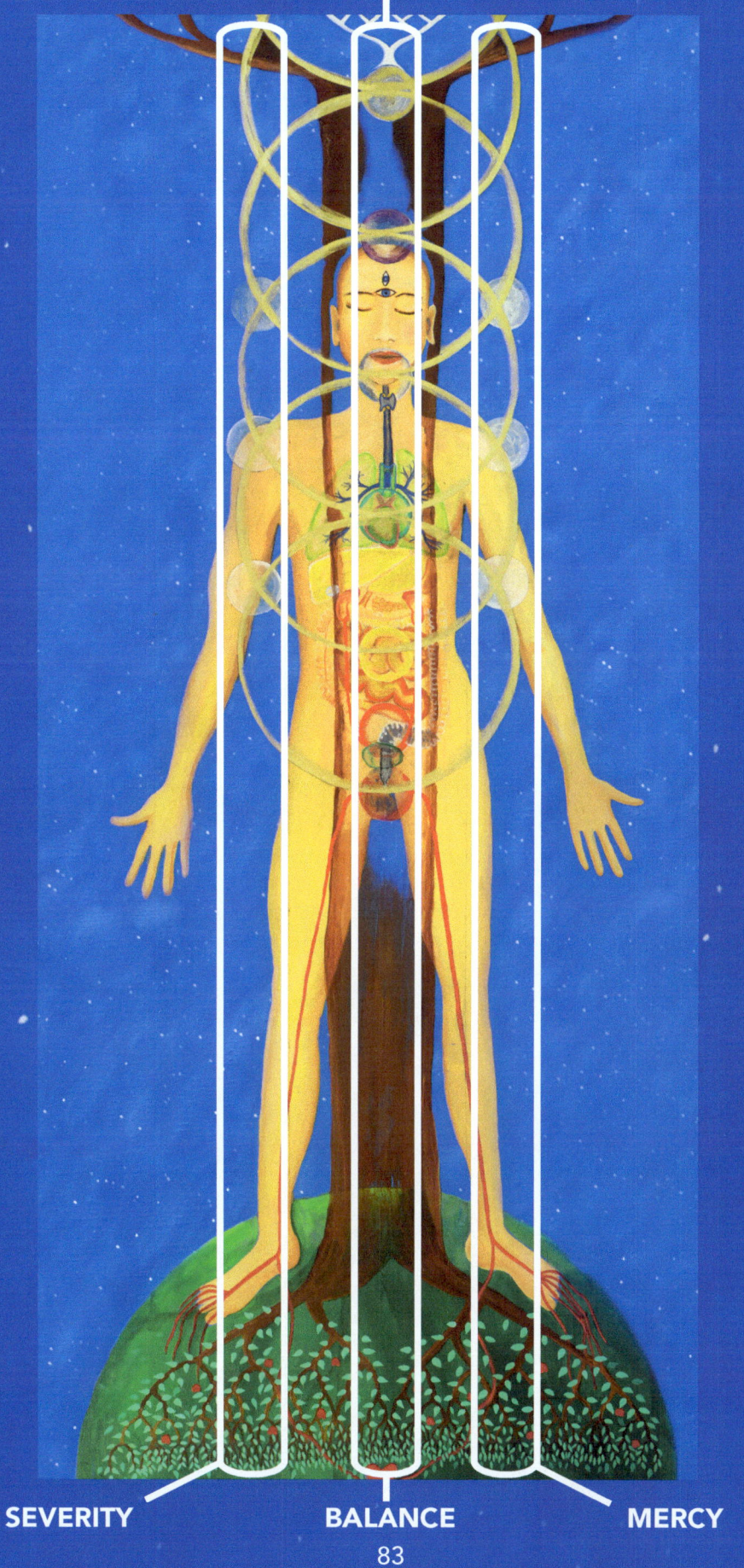

NEUTRAL

SEVERITY   BALANCE   MERCY

THE THREE PILLARS OF LIFE
with Metatron and the Platonic Solids.

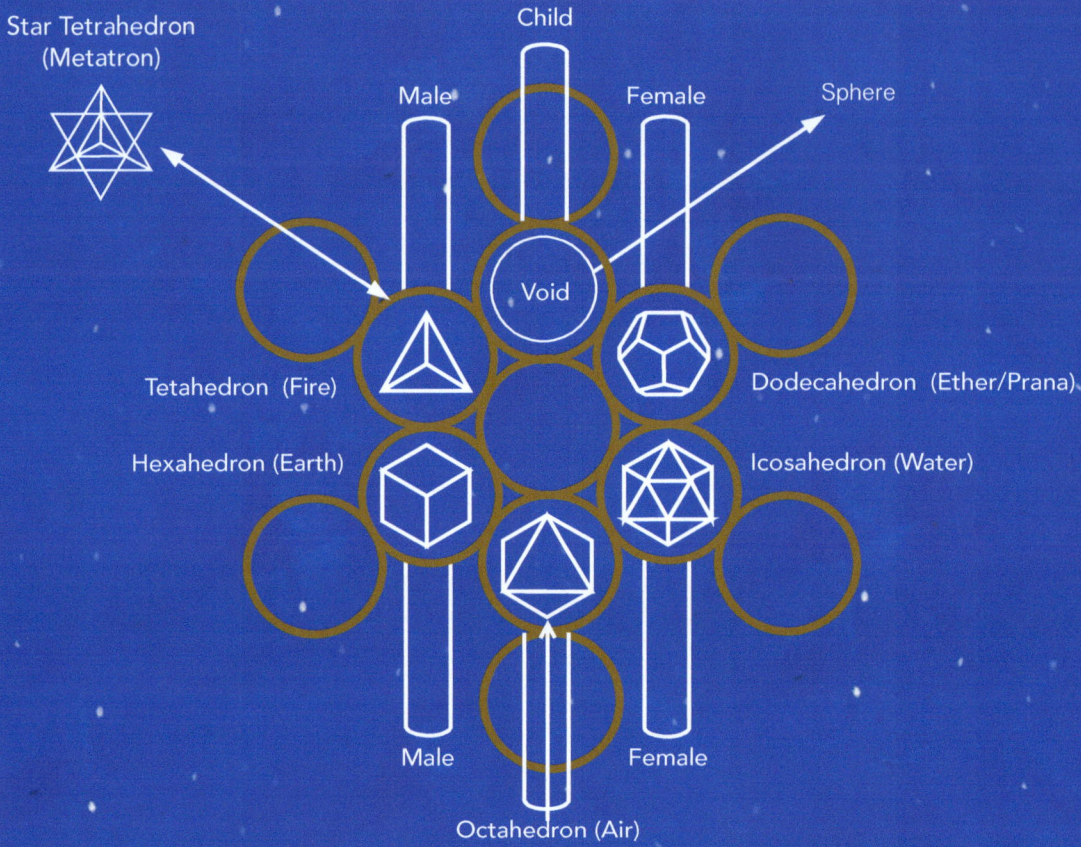

The Pillar of Life explained with the Inverted Tree of Life. (refer to the Kabbalah diagram in the beginning of this section). One of the main premises of the Inverted Tree of Life is the inclusion and position of the ROOT. The Root descends from the VOID or God (ocean) because It has decided to break off, as "a drop from the ocean" and become a soul. The pure soul then descends deeper into matter by incarnating Its Self. This incarnated soul (higher self) is represented by the golden ball under the Root. Between the golden ball and the violet ball exists the auric blueprint fields of subtle light energies that make you YOU. The Root continues to descend to the violet ball (incarnating) as it continues to descend into the crown chakra or Kether (in Kabbalah) into the pineal gland (the vertical third eye), all the way down to the base chakra of the human form.

Our way back to the Void/God/First Source is the reverse, which the Inverted Tree of Life expresses, is the only way to return. The journey back involves the ascension or rising of our energies (kundalini, CHI and prana) up through the spine to the pineal gland, to the golden ball of the incarnated soul, continuing up to the Pure Soul or *the drop of ocean* merging with The Root, the SOURCE or Ocean of All that is. This is the to and from journey of the incarnated soul and some of the main premises of the Inverted Tree of Life.

The premise of the Pillar of Life is the function of the respective pillars: Pillar of Severity, the Pillar of Balance and the Pillar of Mercy. These Pillars represent the nature of this 3D realm, which is polarity and all of the states between the two extreme Pillars. Our task, when we decide to begin our respective journeys, is to return to our point of origin. WE do this when we have found balance or *equanimity* between the two pillars through self-mastery of our body, mind and emotions. We are engaged in a process of remembering, awakening and discovering Who we truly are. We will eventually arrive at our destination with the innocence of a child (center pillar) balanced and in joy. This realization is the reconnection to our already perfect SELF, which is the drop of ocean (pure soul) returning and re-merging with the All (Ocean), God or First Source. "I" merges and is and always has been WE/US/ALL.

INVERTED TREE OF LIFE

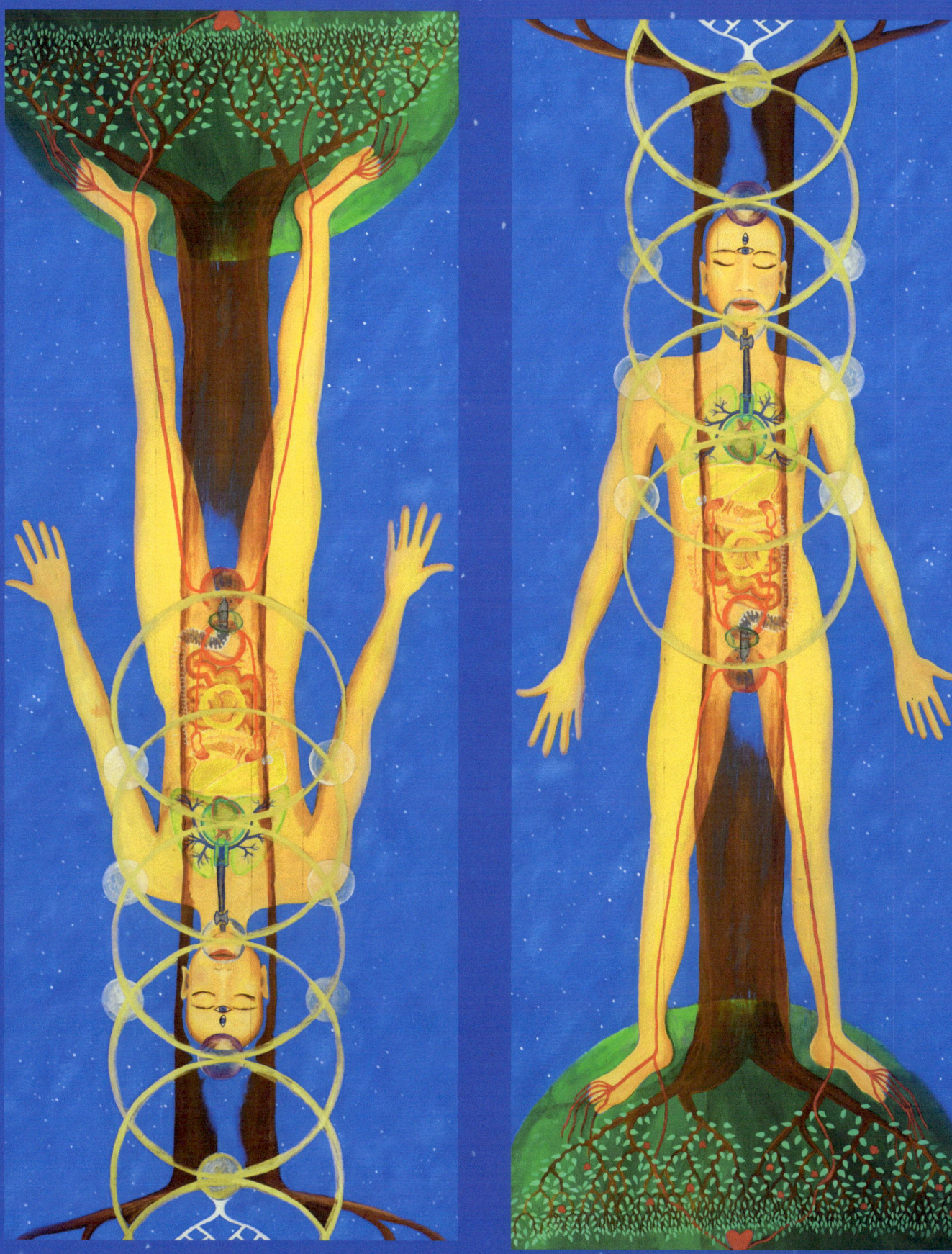

Note: The upright position of the human form with the Root of God descending into the head, gives life to form. How we choose to live and what we do with that *life* either contributes more life or takes life from the planet. Which tree are you?

Significance of the Inverted Tree of Life
and its connection to the Kabbalah and the 13 Sephiroth.
Similar references to the Tree of Life exists in many cultures and spiritual traditions all over the world.

The Inverted Tree of Life and the Kabbalah enhance each other's perspective and positions in the higher realms and the soul's descent into form or matter. The connections to the Divine, as well as the connection to the Earth are included in both. But in the Kabbalah and its 13 Sephiroth, emphasis appears to be more on establishing a reconnection to the Root that originates in the Divine. The Root is *life-giving*, enabling form to literally live as it descends into the human form. Death occurs when the *life-giving* Root connection is severed. How can we and how could we ignore this basic connection?

The Inverted Tree of Life other emphasis appears to be more on one's ability to ground all that the Kabbalah and 13 Sephiroth teach, which is basically intelligence and love in motion. When we can bring down divinity to Earth, it is because we have realized our true self and as a result of that realization, have "spiritualized" all that we do on Earth.

The success, the victory or the glory is represented by each "tree's" or soul's ability to anchor into the Earth what it has manifested or left and or contributed to the Earth. The fullness, the beauty and the fruit of our Tree depend on the choices made and the affects of those choices. What was manifested is a direct result of those choices and what is left behind on Earth and in the Earth's auric fields was and is our individual and collective responsibilities.

"Heaven on Earth" can be realized by our individual and collective intentions and commitment to re-connect to the ROOT and bring down or manifest the Divine. It is our joint free choices and wills that create the heaven or the hell. We are each a tree that individually and collectively contribute. What we contribute is directly reflected back to us. It is what we see in each other and in our world… and we are each responsible for the version of what we see and experience.

What it ALL Means...
inviting the Divine to dwell within you as You.

In my humble opinion, writing this book has brought me to a broader panoramic view of time: past, present and future. It has expanded a deeper meaning and picture of you, me, us and them. It has increased my scope of responsibility and it begins and essentially starts with Self, extends to family, community and the planet at large. It has changed my view of our recent planetary history since the last ice age, roughly between ten and thirteen thousand years ago. Man and our co-created civilizations were and are primarily based on the material world. This material relationship only includes the body and mind. Shamefully, the emotional and spiritual development of Self is lacking and in many cases eliminated or sparsely evident, especially in our institutions, religions and cultures. Our societies are basically only walking on the one leg of mind/body and the other leg has been substituted with a crutch. This crutch really cannot and does not serve at all. We have become delusional thinking that limping with a crutch is walking. But we are not walking, nor skipping, jumping, running or even flying. We are confused and ignorant to feel that this broken method of surviving is thriving. We come into this world already handicapped by the limitation of having access to only ten to twenty percent of our brain capacity. The same exist for the activation of our DNA. In addition to this deficit, we come with a *karmic debt* or *original sin*, based on the past that we have no recollection of. It is increasingly disheartening, when we realize that most of us came back here again and again with NO MEMORIES.

Historically, our very institutions have destroyed, burned, locked up and or denied access to information that our ancestors have dedicatedly left for us. For these mentioned reasons, I am convinced that we are not just reincarnated, but recycled and trapped souls. The continuous delusional "paths" never lead us to liberation, but deeper into an abyss of forgetfulness. Why? We can get stuck on answering that question seemingly forever. I prefer and have learned by this experience, that to just realize these facts, has been enough to motivate me to dig deeper into how we can alter and eventually end this cycle.

The tools in this book provide some ways out. AA (Alcoholics Anonymous) and many self-help groups and institutions offer other ways. All together, there are always a variety of options that lead us within. The depth we travel within will vary. The will and the desire to go the distance, to assume and resume to do anything, remain each person's choice and responsibility. These methods, along with meditation or sitting in the silence to calm your own mind and heart, along with the practice of being the observer and being in the moment (moment to moment); are ways that the *tools* can loosen the grip and release us from the swamp abyss of mind chatter of self and cultural drama.

When we discover and dare to go the distance, there are presents along the way, but only when we are present enough to see and feel them. Space will eventually be created where we will, individually and collectively, connect time: past, present and future. We will All see time as one time. We will realize that we were never separate, but always connected. To "play" the roles well, we had to BELIEVE in our separateness (I/he/she/them/us). This awakening will awaken another and another realization. We will realize that we were the black man and the white man, the rat and the elephant, a dolphin and a starfish, an Israeli and Palestinian, a Hitler and a Gandhi. We all played the sinner and savior alike, the humble master guru and the deceitful priest. We all stole, lied and cheated our neighbors. We all participated in crimes against humanity and our Mother Earth. We were all women, men and children, loved and unloved. We all have been saved and all rescued. We were all warriors for evil and for good. The pendulum has swung from the good, and back to the bad...to and fro countless times. If only we could remember. If only we could recall our wisdom and foolishness. We would then instantly SEE each other and ourselves as Divine and connected. It would instantly halt this nightmarish ego driven movie of disconnectedness and fear. And LOVE would rush in and joyously spread its wonders everywhere!

Language and the Illusion of Separateness

Language can be tricky, specially pronouns, which by their nature divides and distinguishes. Repeated use of these words casts an energetic spell, which solidifies the separateness paradigm. This paradigm contributes to the solidification of aloneness. Over use of I/he/she/me/my/yours and them, validates the separateness paradigm and promotes a perpetual state of perceived non-unification. When we can energetically and intentionally replace I/he/she/it and them with WE and US; we are rupturing the paradigm of separateness. The separateness was and is held together by our collective beliefs and perceptions, which are all based on the illusion of physical manifestation of I/he/she/etc.

We are not considering that beyond manifestation, there exist energetic fields that include thoughts and ideas that seem independent. But these fields do exist in the etheric world, and they are not separate from the physical world. They are actually blueprints that help form the physical world; thought precedes manifestation. Any world that exists is a validation of that connectedness. The universe actually cannot and does not compute disconnection. It only sees One or All. The more we can be and act from the premise of All, the more compassion and empathy can be reflected in the world. There is no separation between others and I, it does not compute. We are. There is only Oneness.

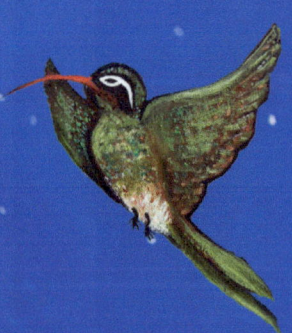

Part 6: Addendum to WOW of the Heart

SeeMore and Matisse have something to add to the "Wow of the Heart" book. These are more practices that will further assist you in developing your meditative or quiet contemplative time.

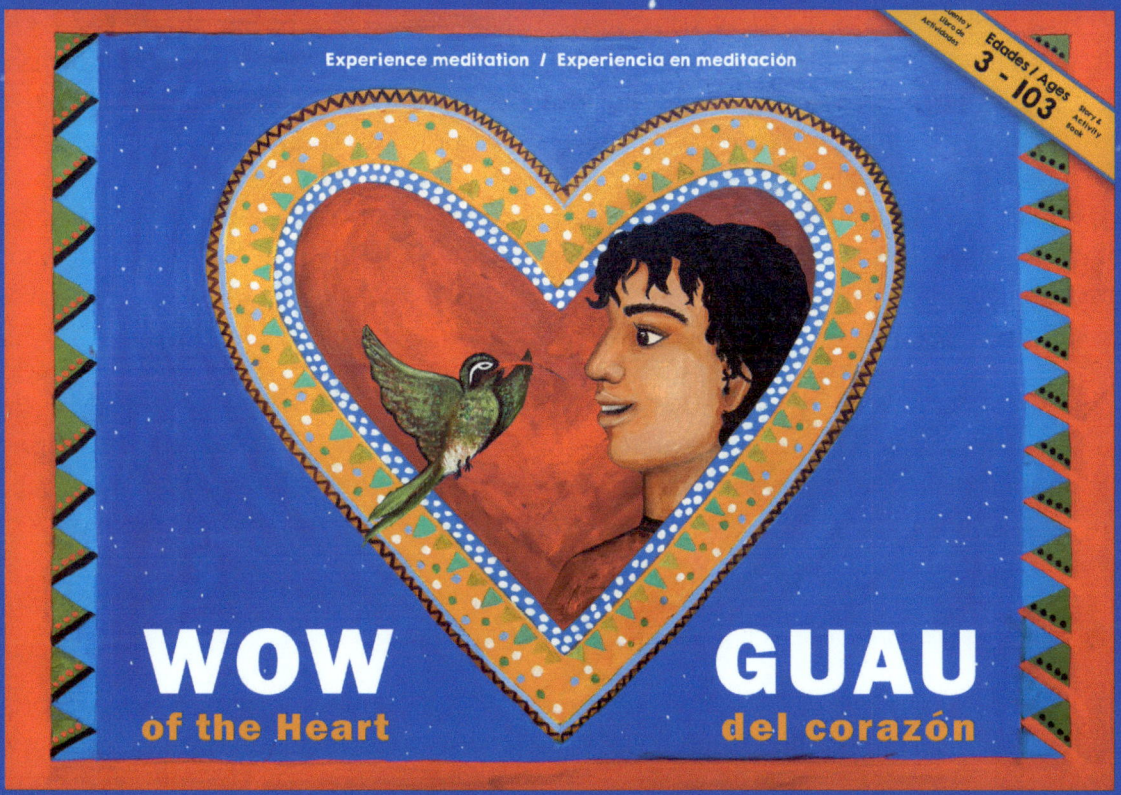

Practices to do along with Meditation

The practices included in this section go along with and reinforce the formal efforts that you make to meditate. Choose the practice that is easiest for you first and add others as you progress.

Practice the Presence. Stop periodically throughout your daily and nightly routines and observe. Go beyond the obvious noises and things in front of you and pay attention and LISTEN to the subtler pulses of life: your heart beat, your breath, the breeze in the trees, a call of a bird in the distance, a loving memory… end these *moments of presence* in gratitude and appreciation.

Practice Truth. We can practice truth by observing and by watching what we are going to say. If what you are going to say is not true, practice refraining from saying it. Start with small non-truths and work your way up…the discipline of tackling the smaller lies will pave an easier road towards living more in truth. Truth is behind the original meaning of the word *kosher*. Truth is the essence of the word *kosher*, in intent and in action and is of the highest value. It is of value, not only from the person that speaks it, but the truth carries a ripple affect out into the community and world. These intentions and actions promote a more truthful paradigm.

Identify a non-desirable habit and try to overcome it. Habits enslave the body and mind to repetitive actions. When these repetitive actions are done without thought and without consciousness they become a habit or an addiction. These actions are *the habit* that is now automatic. These habits are usually not desirable. Gossiping, bullying, over eating, drinking, smoking, drug abuse and excessive attachments to electronics and social media are a few habits/addictions that may take control of you, as opposed to you having control over them. Becoming more conscious of oneself when the habit begins to emerge is the first step in overcoming a potentially bad habit; it helps halt the no thought automatic response. In our current cultural societies, we have *isolated* our selves and have retreated into our own respective worlds. This isolation is much worse for those who have suffered trauma and abuse in childhood and it provides the perfect conditions or atmosphere for habits and addictions to develop. The possibility of this scenario occurring becomes lessened when the trauma and its surrounding and underlying feelings of isolation, abandonment and abuse are dealt with directly. Diving into the Self and investigating the underlying associated feelings is the only way out. Addictions and habits are also a way out, but they never address the issues that are driving one towards the addictive behavior. Choosing to go within and addressing those underlying subtle emotions is actually developing a new habit or coping skill that can directly combat the old bad habit or addiction. Understanding WHY and also how the habit developed can lead one to clues in overcoming habits and the discipline that follows reinforces that self-discovery. These are some of the ways that can empower us and help us regain control over our lives. These actions of healing will integrate within us when we focus on our Self and Nature first, which will lead us out of isolation. As we become healthier, our basis for establishing better relationships with others will also become more successful.

There are many self-help groups that can assist one in overcoming habits and addictions. These groups specialize and are specifically focused to help one to identify, understand and overcome habits/addictions. These are important tools that can lead towards freedom from automatic behaviors. A world without negative habits and addictions is liberating and provides a foundation as it creates space where one's dreams and aspirations can be realized.

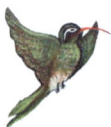 **Pay attention to the diets**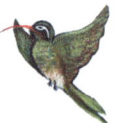

Pay attention to the quality and amount of food and drink you consume. Move in the direction of consuming more water and fresh foods before giving up something… this way makes it easier because more water and more fresh foods naturally wean us from the desire for things that are not so good for us.

Pay attention to your *media diet*. Be aware of the quality of books you read, the films you watch, internet and social media time you spend. Choose subjects that are more inspirational and that validate your POWER.

Pay attention to the content of day dreams and *mind chatter* thinking. Monitor the content of your diet of day dreams and *mind chatter*… if they do not empower you, then start a list of desirable dreams or goals and day dream about manifesting those. You have a choice to choose more worthwhile thoughts that better yourself, family and community.

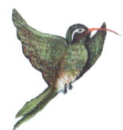 ## Meditation and Equanimity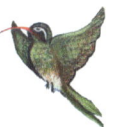

Keep in mind the action to meditate is an action to re-align our self with our higher Self. The road becomes easier if our actions are aligned with our meditative practice and when all aspects of self (the body, mind, emotions and spirit) are moving in the same direction. What slows our progress down are the conflicts that arise between the different aspects of our self. Also the "two steps forward and three steps back" is the other thing that can slow our progress down and keep us in frustration. It will never end until we take the responsibility and stop it. Once we have made the decision to *save* our self first, these new actions will cultivate our confidence and our ability to authentically change, as opposed to half or incomplete changes. This is the only power we truly have. The nature of this dualistic paradigm will not go away, but shifting our lower vibrations into higher vibrations will change the paradigm. These changes in the collective self will minimize the effects of the pendulum and shift us into a state that resonates more in equanimity. This equanimity is our personal and collective salvation, for we have empowered ourselves and are no longer vibrating and resonating with the swing of the pendulum of dualism. Empower yourself by saving yourself through the self-mastery of your bodily and mental habits and live through the higher emotions of spirit. Connect the four parts of you and become the connected YOU… the Divine You.

 ## Author's message to the Youth

This book is not meant to be understood in one reading nor in two or three… remember it is a reference book and you can refer to it as you grow and mature in body, mind, emotions and spirit. Learning is a spiral action. Learning is not a linear action. That is to say that as we "learn" something, we will have experiences that will help make that knowledge more real. In other words, the knowledge will become truer because somehow the experience (s) that you had or have or will have; will validate the feeling of what was learned. It's a fascinating process because many times we do not learn: a, then b, then c, then d… etc. (linear learning). We learn spirally: a, then c, then d, then e, then b, and some times z…it takes time! In spiral learning you will have moments where one piece of information will make other bits of information all come together in one moment and something "clicks" and you will say, "NOW I get it"! Those are "AH HA" moments and they are wonderful! So do not be hard on yourself…always have fun learning and remember it is a continuous process. And lastly, question many things…even this book. Search, find and validate your own answers and make sure that they are genuine… you can feel truth. Remember to be OPEN to other ways of thinking and being and ALWAYS use your imagination…the place and the source of genuine problem solving and ideas!

Remember Einstein? He said, "You can not solve a problem on the same level of thinking in which the problem was created." So genuine answers demand our ability to use our imaginations, to dare and go beyond the same level of a problem. We must meet the challenge and go into the levels that are full of possibilities, where we can truly create, co-create and resolve our dilemmas making the world a better place for ALL.

Bibliography
Combined influences and life study of the following.

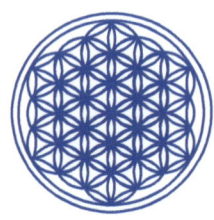

Books/Videos/Films

Anatomy
Leonardo da Vinci Esbozos y dibujos (drawings)   by: Frank Zöllner
The Anatomy Coloring Book by Wynn Kapit and Lawrence M. Elson
Women's Bodies Women's Wisdom by Christiane Northrup M.D.

Heart
- Dr. Carson Wells : world's leading cardiologist, various YouTube/History Channel interviews
- Frank Chester and his studies on the heart. His web site and YouTube lectures.

    - https://youtu.be/1bKJVeIIddU Frank Chester Lecture Sausalito CA 2007   (form (solid) changes the vortex (in water) to double vortex (helix like DNA). Some forms implode the water. Start at 1:20 for the heart)
    - https://youtu.be/ql9kh7L91eg Frank Chester Lecture Seattle Sept 2012 start 1:08 (Projected two cone geometry of the heart of angled layers in motion create other forms triangles to squares and squares back to triangles).
    - Frank Chester from Green Meadow Waldorf School Heart Lecture Series   10/2009 Heart to Chalice/Bell explained especially part 4:

        part 1 start at 2:30 https://youtu.be/eW_URLqFDHs
        part 3 https://youtu.be/LcTiNdKlATU
        part 4 https://youtu.be/egtC8OfDk7I geometric heart forms.. (2:20 goes from chestrahedron to a chalice or bell form when spinning in water).

Frequency, Energy and Healing
- Nicolas Tesla, books, lectures, YouTubes.
- Quantum Healing by Deepak Chopra
- Dr. Bruce Lipton: The Biology of Belief * and various lectures
- Hands of Light by Barbara Ann Brennan
- Dan Winter, YouTube lectures
- www.HeartMath.com
- Dr. Joe Dispensa: You are the Placebo,   various lectures and studies*
- The Power of Now *by Eckhart Tolle
- Nassin Haramein: Physicist: various lectures
- The Holographic Universe by Michael Talbot
- AA's The 12 Steps A Way Out
- Masaru Emoto: studies on water... how intention/consciousness affects water (crystals).
- Eric Rankin   https://youtu.be/FY74AFQl2qQ   www.SonicGeometry.com
- Sonic Geometry: The Language of Frequency and Form parts 1 and 2
- FOR REAL FUN watch CYMATICS: Science vs. Music by Niguel Stanford YOUTUBE (he shows how vibration, frequency with sand, water, fire, and even electricity respond to SOUND!!!!

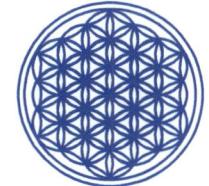

Ancient Archeology, the Kabbalah and other Ancient Wisdom Teachings
- The Spiritual Essence of Man, Master Choa Kok Sui (The 13 Point Kabbalah)
  Thank you Master Choa Kok Sui
- The Ancient Secrets of the Flower of Life vol.1 and 2 by Drunvalo Melchizedek
- Michael Tellinger and Graham Hancock ancient archeology, YouTube
- Egyptian School of Mystery, various you tubes and lectures.
- Nicolas Tesla's Ghost, YouTubes lectures Randall Carlson
- Bright Insight: YouTube lectures By researcher Jimmy

Eastern Thought and Paradigm Shifting
- Autobiography of a Yogi and Man's Eternal Quest. Self Realization Fellowship: various and numerous other books and lectures* by Parmahansa Yogananda
- Tibetan Buddhism (especially Dzogchen Yoga)
- The Tibetan Book of Living and Dying* by Sogyal Rinpoche),
- Greg Braden: The Divine Matrix, You Tube: The 7 Essene Mirrors*, various other lectures
- Anastasia and The Ringing Cedar Series Books 1-4 by Vladimir Megre
- Walter Russell: incredible drawings/charts depicting the secrets of the universe.
- 20 years of mentorship with Monk Brother Turiyananda of SRF
- Sri Ramana Maharshi

Other: includes film, web sites, lectures etc.
- Wingmakers, web site www.wingmakers.com
- Avatar (the film by James Cameron)
- The Game (film with Michael Douglas and Sean Penn)
- Contact: Robert Zemeckis, Director.
- Samadhi, Part 1 and 2 by Daniel Schmidt.
- Matrix Trilogy, V for Vendetta and Cloud Atlas films by The Wachowskis
- www.suspiciousobservers.org
- https://youtu.be/Fbyc9JW3vtk
    Randy Powell: Intro to Vortex Math Part 1 of 2
- https://youtu.be/fEE55gcttqo
    Randy Powell: Intro to Vortex Math Part 2 of 2

- my own inner guidance, intuition and lucid dreams.
- Mexican culture: conducive for opening the heart.
- my family, friends and acquaintances that gave me the opportunities: to discover, to practice and to implement those realizations that awakened and continue to awaken me to my truer Self. They helped me on my road, to become a better person.

Author's note: There are no exact page numbers that I am capable of specifying, as each book and lecture in it's respective context, along with my state of mind and being at the time of reading (s) changed and evolved. It is not adequate and would not do justice to these valuable works to separate any of its portions; it would diminish the significance of the whole.

Thank you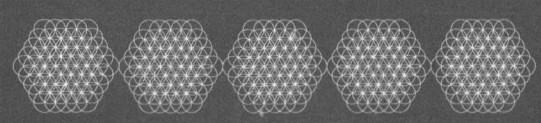

To those who worked on the book…
Firstly, I like to thank Jorge Luis Monteverde Torres for his outstanding contribution; the graphic design, diagrams and his expertise and assistance with the layout added immensely to this project. He also edited the Spanish version and contributed to editing the English version.
Jorge's personal dedication in search of his own truth merged with his professional life. He made himself a living example. His sincere efforts and enthusiasm added a proficiency to this project and made it more magical. I truly felt and feel blessed and privileged that such an angel like person assisted me with this book, a labor of love.

Gratitude to Tom Berridge for being one of the first editors that got us moving right direction. A huge thank you to Claude Vogel for his photography and his wife Celia Vasquez for their long lasting friendship and support. Claudia Kane was extremely helpful in editing portions of the English version, which contributed greatly to the Spanish version. Her constant support and encouragement is highly cherished and greatly appreciated. I could not have completed it without her.

To family and more friends…
As I watch the little ones grow and see the world that they must deal with, I realize that it is imperative that we address our emotional maturity and responsability to self and community. As we evolve and nurture the self that dwells within, we are empowered to manifest our best qualities. So I thank all children. Your combined inspiration motivates me to accomplish this commitment. May all children, including the child within every adult, find some comfort and answers in this book that will assist with the journey into Self, discovering that God dwells within you as You.

No work of art is possible without the love and support of family and friends.
Special thank you to Azia Coffman H. and Luis Arroyo for being HERE during this endeavor and for your day-to-day invaluable love and support. Coy Coffman H., I thank you for your diligence and love. You "never give up" and inspire me to do the same. Special thank you to Marc Hayles Dunn and Suzanne Demas for showing me that knowing something intellectually without the all important added emotional knowledge (that many times gets buried); is by-passing one of the most powerful inter-connecting parts of who we are; the part that enables us to actually "move the mountain." Thanks for digging deep… it gave this book more "backbone." A thousand thank you (s) to family and friends near and far but always in the heart: Erik and Marla Caesar, Bert Hayles, Becky Silva, Tom Stansberry, Mary Vernieu, Ross Vail, Eleanor Andrews, Susan Carol, Octavio López, Cynthia Torres, Jessica Flood, Nick Papadopoulos, Cathy Buchanan, Howard Ekman, Tina Allen and Brother Turiyananda. Also a huge thank you to the owner and staff of Valle de la Paz in Valle de Bravo for creating a place of true extraordinary wonder. Dieter le Noir and Yolanda Suarez del Real, by their living and day to day examples have inspired me to "go the distance" by what they and others have co-created at Valle la Paz. Lastly (and firstly) a humble deep bow for the never ending support, blessings and love from Paramahansa Yogananda and Sri Yukteswar Giri.

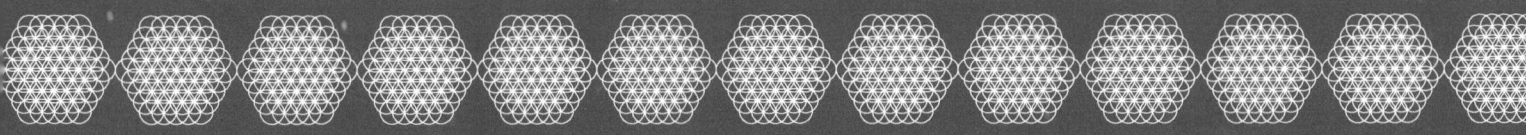

About the Author

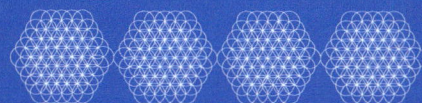
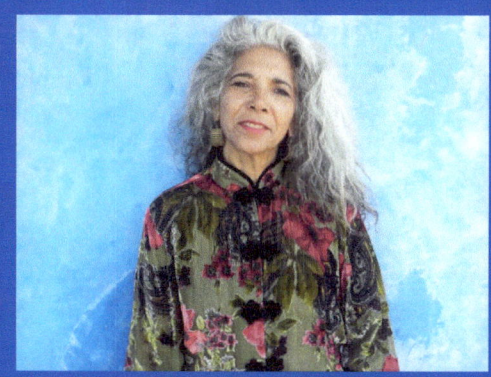

Nanette E. Hayles is an educator, author and self taught artist. She resides in a small town in Mexico. She is dedicated to self-knowledge that encourages and validates one's own unique experiences as an individual's way to self realize. In addition to our own self-respect for our unique journeys into self, we must also extend that same courtesy and respect to others and their paths. Eventually these journeys will lead us all to the same discovery and inner peace… that we are ALL unique versions of the same Truth.

This book is a part of the "Matisse and SeeMore WOW Series" and it is dedicated to these same goals. "Wow of the Heart" is the first book and it is about meditation and is bilingual. "Wow of the Magical Body" is the second book and it is available in both English and Spanish. The third book will be released in 2021.

"Children" of all ages are never too young or too old to awaken and empower one's own divinity by questioning, searching and validating our unique experiences. When we know THYSELF, we heal thyself and when we heal thyself, we collectively heal each other and our world.

Book 3 in 2021…this time a magical story.

"When the power of love overcomes the love of power, the world will know the peace".
Jimi Hendrix

"If we could read the secret history of our enemies, we would find enough sorrow and suffering to disarm all of our hostility".
Henry Longfellow

About the Art

Original art "The Magical Body" by: Nanette E. Hayles. Diagrams/enhancements/cropping and other manipulation of images: Jorge Luis Monteverde Torres with Nanette E. Hayles. Photo credit: Claude Vogel.

Dates: 2013-2016   **Size:** 4'x 8' (122 cm x 244 cm)   **Medium:** Oil on wood

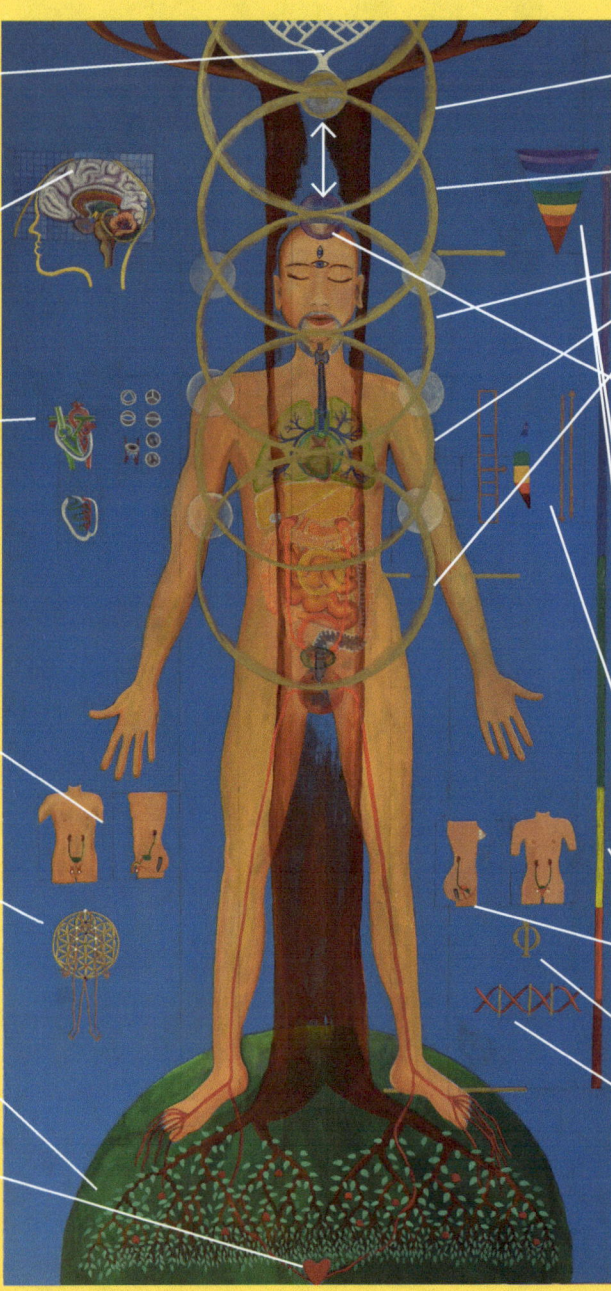

1. Root/God/First Source.

2. Brain (side view) follows the basic Fibonacci spiral and sequence forms.

3. The heart and its vortexes and valves.

4. Male human form.

5. Kabbalah and the Sephiroth (13) overlaid over the Flower of Life symbol.

6. Tree branches and leaves are fractals.

7. Heart (pulse) center of Mother Earth.

1. Five Golden (inner) rings/spheres of the Flower of Life pattern = 3D realm/material world. The sixth ring/sphere=ascension into the next realm (astral).

2. Space between the golden small globe and violet globe= the etheric field which contain the mental, emotional and spiritual blueprints of YOU.

3. Frequency and the emotions.

4. Spectrums: visible and invisible (electromagnetic).

5. Female human form.

6. PHI (Greek) symbol.

7. DNA strand and PHI proportion AND The 2 meter rainbow bar=the total length of one complete DNA strand.

This art piece was conceived to be as user friendly as possible, which the Naïve art style accomplishes. The hope was to create an atmosphere of fun and curiosity in viewing the human form. Almost every theme covered in the book is on this four-foot by eight-foot art image. All other art images are from "WOW of the Heart" and other series of artwork by the author with photo credit to Howard Ekman.

The Other 80-90% is WOW

To come all this way, to descend in to form and experience LIFE …and to not challenge nor go the distance and search within…to at least awaken a portion of the 80 to 90% of our minds and DNA…is like mistaking a beautiful precious diamond, for a piece of common glass and throwing it into the sea.

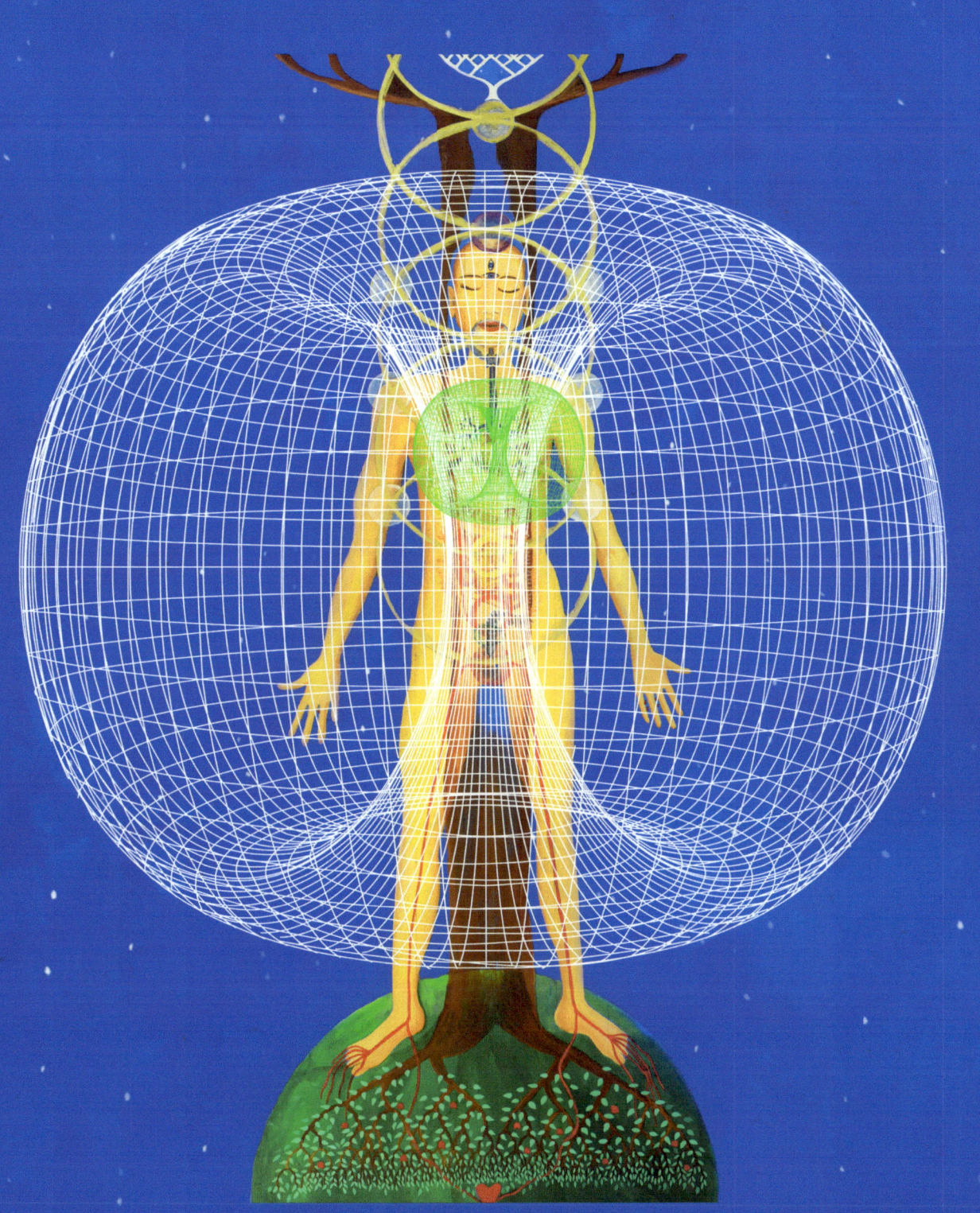

www.ingramcontent.com/pod-product-compliance
Lightning Source LLC
Chambersburg PA
CBHW041432010526
44118CB00002B/56